"Professor Henderson has, from different angles, examined the 'conventional wisdom' that residential care for children and youth is *inherently* harmful to their development. He concludes that this 'wisdom' is scientifically completely unsustainable. As professionals (in training), policymakers and scientists, we have been enriched with a very convincing book."

Erik J. Knorth, *Professor, University of Groningen, the Netherlands*

"This text fills an important gap in the literature on residential care. It offers significant new analyses based on an extensive review of relevant literature. This challenge to the 'conventional wisdom' is overdue and a critically important addition to the literature."

James P. Anglin, *PhD, Emeritus Professor, University of Victoria*

"A must-read corrective to conventional wisdom on residential child care. Henderson provides valuable analysis and perspective that will help to shape a more nuanced view of residential child care policy, research and practice."

James K. Whittaker, *PhD, Charles O. Cressey Endowed Professor of Social Work Emeritus, The University of Washington*

"Highly vulnerable children often fail in foster homes, retraumatized by multiple placements. Some require intensive relational care, turning trauma into resilience. Henderson's well-researched book deflates fake science that is eliminating the most intensive alternatives for these young people."

Larry K. Brendtro, *PhD, Author, Reclaiming Youth at Risk: Futures of Promise*

"This scholarly exploration of research on group care for vulnerable children crosses years and continents. The forensic approach to the knowledge base will be welcomed by all who argue for a continuing place for good quality children's homes within the range of placements for (older) children."

June Thoburn, *CBE, LiitD, MSW, Emeritus Professor of Social Work, University of East Anglia*

Challenging the Conventional Wisdom about Residential Care for Children and Youth

Is residential care "inherently harmful"? This book argues that this conventional wisdom is wrong and is, itself, harmful to a significant number of children and youth.

The presumptive view is based largely on overgeneralizations from research with infants and very young children raised in extremely deprived environments. A careful analysis of the available research supports the use of high-quality residential care as a treatment of choice with certain groups of needy children and youth, not a last resort intervention. The nature of high-quality care is explored through child development theory and research and two empirically supported models of care are described in detail.

It will be of interest to all scholars and students of child development, child welfare, youth work, social work, and education as well as professionals working within these fields.

Bruce B. Henderson is Professor Emeritus of Psychology at Western Carolina University. He received his doctorate from the University of Minnesota's Institute of Child Development and is a member of the Society for Research in Child Development. He has published widely on children's curiosity, memory development, and higher education.

Routledge Advances in Social Work

Using Art for Social Transformation
International Perspective for Social Workers, Community Workers and Art Therapies
Edited by Eltje Bos and Ephrat Huss

Revitalising Critical Reflection in Contemporary Social Work Research, Practice and Education
Edited by Christian Franklin Svensson and Pia Ringø

The Body Politics of Glocal Social Work
Essays on the Post-Anthropocentric Condition
Mona B. Livholts

Language Discordant Social Work in a Multilingual World
The Space Between
Hilde Fiva Buzungu

Social Work, Social Welfare and Social Development in Nigeria
A Postcolonial Perspective
Mel Gray and Solomon Amadasun

International Perspectives on Parenting Support and Parental Participation in Children and Family Services
Edited by Carmel Devaney and Rosemary Crosse

Against Critical Thinking in Health, Social Care and Social Work
Reframing Philosophy for Professional Practice
Tom Grimwood

Challenging the Conventional Wisdom about Residential Care for Children and Youth
A Good Place to Grow
Bruce B. Henderson

Challenging the Conventional Wisdom about Residential Care for Children and Youth

A Good Place to Grow

Bruce B. Henderson

Routledge
Taylor & Francis Group
LONDON AND NEW YORK

First published 2024
by Routledge
4 Park Square, Milton Park, Abingdon, Oxon OX14 4RN

and by Routledge
605 Third Avenue, New York, NY 10158

Routledge is an imprint of the Taylor & Francis Group, an informa business

British Library Cataloguing-in-Publication Data
A catalogue record for this book is available from the British Library

ISBN: 978-1-032-56473-9 (hbk)
ISBN: 978-1-032-56478-4 (pbk)
ISBN: 978-1-003-43570-9 (ebk)

DOI: 10.4324/9781003435709

Typeset in Sabon
by codeMantra

To the children, youth, and families at the Black Mountain Home and to the staff members who care for them with unconditional love.

Contents

Acknowledgment

I thank Professor Heidi Buchanan for reading the entire manuscript and the others at Hunter Library who were so helpful tracking resources, even during a pandemic. The editors and authors of the chapters in *Revitalizing Residential Care for Children and Youth* provided me with a useful global perspective. Martha Holden was encouraging at a key time, and her CARE team is a model of good practice. Jim Anglin was unceasingly supportive throughout the research and writing process. Having access to his vast expertise provided me with a secure base for exploration. I cannot give him enough credit. I thank Cheryl and Tom Campbell for showing me how residential care should be done, with a selfless devotion to children and youth who have experienced too little love and attention in their short lives. And, it was Judy, my rock in all of life, who got me to care about children in residential care in the first place.

1 Challenging the Conventional Wisdom

This book conflicts with the *Zeitgeist*. It will make some readers angry. It challenges beliefs that are strongly held by many people who genuinely care about children and youth. There will be those who cannot believe that what I say is true. It is important that I make my argument as clear as possible. I will start with the book's title.

The Conventional Wisdom about Residential Care

Here are the essential characteristics of the conventional wisdom about residential care for children and youth (this is conventional wisdom in the anglophone countries but often not in continental western Europe and elsewhere):

Assumption 1. Residential care of all types is an inherently bad form of care.

- a Residential care is necessarily institutional and routinized rather than relational and individualized;
- b Residential care is necessarily operationalized using shift care workers with a high instance of turnover who do not provide consistent care;
- c Children and youth do not develop relationships with adults in residential care;
- d Children and youth learn negative behaviors from their peers in residential care;
- e Residential care is not only inferior care; it causes actual psychological damage to children and youth.

Assumption 2. Because of assumption 1, residential care should only be used as a last resort or even eliminated (as made explicit most recently in the Lancet Group Commission Report of 2020, Goldman et al., 2020). Foster care is always superior to residential care.

Assumption 3. Assumptions 1 and 2 are based on a substantial body of research with children of all ages, across the world. It is this research that has led to calls by several professional organizations to minimize or

DOI: 10.4324/9781003435709-1

even eliminate residential care for dealing with children and youth who cannot live with their families of origin.

Assumption 4. Residential care is too expensive and always more expensive than other forms of care.

This conventional wisdom is held by those at the United Nations concerned with children, by the staff at the Annie E. Casey Foundation, by the Board of Directors of the American Orthopsychiatric Association (now the Global Alliance for Behavioral Health and Social Justice), by the members of the Lancet Group Commission on Deinstitutionalisation, and by other organizations and scholars in the United States and across the world. The point of my book is to challenge each of the assumptions of this conventional wisdom by examining the available research literature relevant to them. Challenging the conventional wisdom is important because as an anonymous reviewer of an early version of this book so cogently put it:

> ...the 'story' that group care is harmful... is harmful [itself] because it drives funding, policies, legislation, and services without an evidence base. This book has consolidated the evidence (or lack thereof) about what we actually know about providing out-of-home care for children so that decisions can be made based on what we know versus ideological and economic decisions.

Those who hold to the conventional wisdom claim children of all ages and personal histories should be in families. Biological families preferably; adoptive or foster if necessary. Never in an "institution." Although I believe the family is normally fundamental to children's development, especially the development of infants and young children, I also believe the conventional wisdom about residential care is wrong for a significant number of children and youth. I did not know that when I started this project. I personally knew individual children and youth for whom residential care had not been harmful, indeed had changed their lives for the better. I did not know if those were unusual cases. As a trained research child psychologist, I was inclined to go to the available data. Over the past three years, I have done so. I am now prepared to challenge the conventional wisdom, not based on the ideological positions of agencies, commissions, or pundits, or anecdotal evidence from passionate witnesses, but based on a careful, analytic review of the available research literature.

A Good Place to Grow

In various venues and reports, organizations and individuals who hold to the conventional wisdom have claimed that residential settings are "no place to grow up." My title conveys that for some children and youth a period in residential care can provide an opportunity to flourish. The conventional wisdom gets applied to children of all ages. The United Nations Convention on the Rights of the Child defines "children" as those under 18. Most states in the United States do not license residential care for children under five years of age except for short periods during an emergency (e.g., when very young children are suddenly removed from a home, usually by law enforcement, because they are in imminent danger). In well-developed child welfare systems, residential care is one component in a system of care that includes foster care, adoption, and independent living programs. Most children between the ages of five and ten who require out-of-home care will spend a short period in residential care or go directly into foster care. As we will see, the research on infants and very young children in residential care has been inappropriately generalized to older children. Yet there are good reasons for placing children between five and ten years of age in high-quality residential care for a time, including to keep sibling groups together and for children who have already experienced the instability of multiple foster placements. Children under ten, in rare cases, may need time to grow in the environment provided by good residential care. They do not need to "grow up" there, but the time there can and will allow them to develop and make it more likely they will experience successful fostering, adoption, or reunification with their family of origin.

Residential care has become an option of "last resort" for children and youth in the United States, Canada, the United Kingdom, and other countries, not because research has shown it to be ineffective or harmful, but because of the overgeneralization of research findings on infants and very young children from extremely deprived environments. My fear is not that effective residential care will no longer receive governmental funding except in highly unusual circumstances. That has already happened (in the United States, through the Family First Prevention Services Act of 2018). Residential care across the world is literally cancelled out in the view of the future in Figure 4 on page 617 of Goldman et al., 2020, a position statement from a prestigious source. My fear is that those who know how effective high-quality residential care can be for those it best fits will no longer be permitted to offer it.

Those who call for the end of residential care are doing so out of admirable motives. I think they are mistaken. I would not go as far as Fulcher (2009) who charges that those who want to eliminate residential care are "...so-called scholars who have never, ever worked with troubled or troublesome children and young people in residential care" (Fulcher, 2009, p. vi). But there may be some truth to what Fulcher goes on to say about the critics: "Rarely have they listened to life stories told by those who have found respite, solace, opportunities and emotional commitment through relationships offered through positive residential care experiences" (Fulcher, 2009, p. vi). Regardless, I offer the argument provided in this book as an alternative way to think about residential care.

An International Problem

Residential care is an issue everywhere. There are children and youth who need support outside their families, at least for a time, and sometimes for a long time, all over the world. In a recent and important book, an august set of editors who have studied residential care for decades, Whittaker, Holmes, del Valle, and James (2023b), present chapters about children's welfare and residential care in 16 different countries. The conclusion of that book (Whittaker, Holmes, del Valle, & James, 2023a) suggests some general international trends regarding residential care: (a) increasing concern with the quality of care, including increasing qualifications for direct care staff and using "evidence-based" practices; (b) development of specialized care for high-need children and youth; (c) increasing use of foster care; (d) increased focus on continuing family engagement and envisioning of being able to quickly and safely intervene with and reunify families; (e) adapting residential care for dealing with unaccompanied migrant children, especially in European countries; (f) a move to smaller units of residential care; and (g) more concern for working with youth through the transition to adulthood.

In contrast to these commonalities, among the major differences across countries is the extent to which residential care is respected and utilized. Some continental European countries use residential care at a high level, whereas the anglophone countries, including the United States, have the lowest utilization of residential care, with a strong preference for foster care when families break down. It may not be coincidental that the anglophone countries are those where there have been especially unsettling histories of dealing with indigenous children and youth. Some countries have enacted laws limiting the use of residential care in any individual case but routinely violate those laws (Whittaker et al., 2023b). But as we will see, there are calls from international groups to eliminate the use of residential care entirely.

Much of the research reviewed in this book has been conducted in North America and Europe, but there are studies from five continents. The central dilemma is the same across nations. Is there something inherently harmful about residential care or can residential care provide one positive environment for children in need? The day-to-day complexities of finding homes for children and youth around the developing world are beyond the scope of this book. The international movement toward closing "institutions" (large, impersonal, unstimulating environments) for infants and very young children is a good idea. It also only makes sense to cease practices that are counterproductive like those of the "orphanage industry" and "orphanage tourism" (e.g., Rotabi, Roby, & Bunker, 2017) that purport to support such institutions. However, the "how" of finding stable, resourced families for older children and youth from across the developing world is less clear to me.

Many of the policy statements from agencies and foundations equate "family" with unalloyed good and "institution" with unalloyed bad. As a child psychologist, I find it hard to understand the relative ease implied in new legislation and policy of fixing the family problems of neglect, abuse, alcohol and drugs, chronic mental instability, fundamental family dysfunction, and criminality. I find it hard to understand the uncritically rosy picture of family reunification, foster care, and adoption inherent in the simplistic "family as good" contrast with residential care. Perhaps like Fulcher, I am left wondering if the researchers and policy makers, the professors of social work, medicine, and psychology, who propose this simple contrast of family versus residential care have spent more than a few moments dealing with the complex child welfare cases like those I have witnessed over the past 30 years in my small part of the world. Surely, they do not read biographies. Certainly, they are not listening to voices of educated former foster care children like those in Brown and Seita's (2009) volume. Even if they did, those stories would have limited value. Testimonies about individual experiences can and should enrich our understanding of the issues. However, you can find testimonies to praise or condemn *any* kind of care. The purpose of this book is to weigh the academic research on forms of residential care, with all its flaws, for and against residential care, not to engage in memoir wars.

Historical Perspectives on the "Last Resort"

I am not going to provide a comprehensive history of residential care. I will use history when it helps contextualize specific issues (e.g., in the section in Chapter 3 on institutions). A good beginning of a history has been made elsewhere and I refer you to those sources (e.g., Anglin & Brendtro, 2017; Courtney & Hughes-Heuring, 2009; Doroshow, 2019; English, 1984; Higginbotham, 2017; Jones, 1993; McKenzie, 2009; Smith, 1995; Smith, 2009), but do watch out for histories that lack context and nuance (e.g., MacLean, 2003). However, I will make a few comments about how residential care became the option of last resort in so many countries. First, it is important to note that the extant sites of residential care in developed countries cannot be compared to those of 40 or even 20 years ago. The typical residential treatment centers and children's homes of today have many of the characteristics of high-quality care I present in Chapter 6.

The decline in the use of residential care and its position as an option of last resort, especially in anglophone countries, has had much more to do with economics and the climate of opinion than with research evidence and that has been the case for many years (Clough, 2005; Knorth & Harder, 2023). Among other factors that have led to residential care being seen as the last resort, three seem particularly important. First, some old institutions of the past were simply horrible places for children. The scandals associated with real, inexcusable physical and sexual abuse, even if they represent a small minority of institutions, put individual organizations in a bad light (Doroshow, 2019) and have continued to do so (Gilligan, 2023). The accounts of the egregious efforts to de-culture indigenous children and youth who should never have been removed from their families in North America (e.g., Stout,

2012; Woolford, 2015) and Australia (Jacobs, 2006), for example, going back to the 19th century in some places, are devastating. Although scandals of abuse and neglect have applied to all places where children live, including foster homes and families of origin, the stories about institutions that purportedly were designed to protect children are especially memorable because they so betray a commitment to helping children.

Second, there are social scientists and practitioners who are convinced that all children and youth should be raised in families, typically conceived of as traditional nuclear families. This ideology is apparent in debates about residential care as early as at the White House Conference of 1909. The conference's final resolution stated that "Home life is the highest and finest product of civilization...children should not be deprived of it except for urgent and compelling reasons" (*Proceedings of the White House Conference on the Care of Dependent Children*, 1909, p. 192). The conferees sensibly concluded that simple conditions of poverty were not such a reason. The conferees also cited the prison-like conditions of many orphanages of the 19th century and recommended the "cottage plan" to replace institutions but favored foster care when out-of-home care was needed. Later in the 20th century, concerns about residential care for children and youth were included in the deinstitutionalization movement (see Chapter 3) that influenced the closing of mental hospitals (Geller, 2000), state schools for the mentally disabled (Goode, Hill, Reiss, & Bronston, 2013; Trent, 2016), prisons and juvenile detention facilities (Millham, Bullock, & Cherrett, 1975), and other "total institutions" in Goffman's (1961) terms.

Third, and perhaps most germane to the arguments in this book, scientists focused on the theoretical nature-nurture issue and the effects of early experience have used studies of children in residential care, specifically infants in institutional care, to support their side or deflate the opposition. Many of the classic studies about residential care described in Chapter 2 of this book were and are used in nature-nurture debates. If nurture is crucial in development, children reared in deprived environments will not develop normally because they were not evolutionarily prepared to deal with unexpected (i.e., abnormal) experiences (King, Humphreys, & Gotlib, 2019). If, on the other hand, children are not greatly influenced by their environments because they are prepared by evolution to respond adaptively to wide variation in environments, they may be resilient in the face of deprivation. Unless the deprivation is extreme indeed or is very long lasting. Classic studies of orphanages (e.g., Skeels, 1966 and see Wolins, 1974) often were optimistic about interventions that could help children recover from early environmental deprivation. Modern studies of extreme deprivation, like those described in Chapter 4, have led to the conclusion that when infants are deprived of early reciprocal interactions, they are not likely to develop normally. However, the nature-nurture issue has proved to be much more complex than these studies suggest, involving questions of epigenesis, the nature of environments, and the plasticity of the human brain (e.g., Flynn, 2016; Goldhaber, 2012; Lock & Palsson, 2016).

This Book

I am challenging the conventional wisdom hostile to residential care in this book. I do not come to this task as an insider. During a four-decade academic career I never engaged the child welfare literature, but my academic credentials and experience are related. My research on children focuses on the development of curiosity and exploratory behavior and on memory development. My ventures into the applied world focused on issues in public schools and day cares and on pedagogical and policy issues in higher education. None of my hundred or so publications appear in child welfare journals. However, for engaging the residential care literature I have found that my background prepared me well. Training in research methodology, child development theory, and knowledge about parent and peer relationships all are relevant to the study of children and youth in the welfare system.

I do not intend to be defensive. Those who support high-quality residential care have been too defensive. However, let me be clear again about what I am *not* saying. First, not all family-less children and youth should be in residential care. Residential care is not for infants or young children except in emergencies. High-quality residential care should be available for older children and adults as one option among many. It should be a matter of fit. What setting provides the most resources and stability for a particular individual (or sibling groups)? Children and youth should not be in residential care just because their families are poor. Second, I am not saying all residential care is good. Poor residential care exists and should not (Wang, 2016). We can describe quality care and we should continue to develop standards that would lead to the elimination of poor care. Third, I am not arguing that high-quality childcare is cheap. It is not. However, when needed, the expense should be undertaken. Fourth, I do not believe high-quality residential care is easy to do. It is not. But it also is not impossible. We can use the existing positive exemplars as models and provide good care for those who need it. Finally, I am not saying that we know everything we need to know. We know much too little about child-environment correspondences that lead to optimal development, how to train people to provide good care, or just what factors make children and youth emotionally and educationally resilient.

In Chapter 2, I will use two illustrations to introduce the main themes of the book. Both show how positions on residential care have been based on research inadequate to justify the elimination of residential care for children and youth. Chapter 3 provides a primer on some of the conceptual and methodological concerns that help map out the issues in the research literature reviewed in the rest of the book. In Chapter 4, I will survey portions of the research that I believe have misled many scholars and practitioners to judge residential care to be bad practice, led to the conventional wisdom. While it is clear is that extremely deprived environments are harmful for infants and young children, a very limited set of research findings has been inappropriately overgeneralized across varied forms of care, varied ages, and children and youth with very different needs. Chapter 5 will selectively review the research that could have shown residential care to be harmful, but, instead, supports the use of residential care as part of an array of services. The quality of care is more important than its site. For some young people, residential care provides their greatest chance to thrive, a good place to grow. I will argue in Chapter 6 that quality residential care can be defined, already has been, and does exist. Chapter 7 includes detailed descriptions of a two programmatic instantiations of quality care that deserve broad dissemination. I will conclude in Chapter 8 with a set of propositions gleaned from my reading of the residential literature of the past 30 years or so.

A central issue in this book is whether research shows that residential care should be a last resort or whether it offers an optimal environment for some children and youth. Those on both sides of the issue are motivated by concerns for the welfare of children and youth. But we need to do more than care about children's welfare. We need to demonstrate our care by finding those means by which they will best thrive. The dirty secret (and it is not even that much of a secret) of the child welfare industry around the world is the number of different places children and youth have had to live in during their young lives. For too many children and youth, adoption has not been an option or has not worked. For too many children and youth, foster care has solved no problems. I am convinced that the unconscionable number of placements many children and youth suffer through is due in large part to a concern with a "least restrictive environment" that has overridden the fundamental need of children and youth for stability, restricting their experience of their environments in the worst possible ways. Too many of the calls to cancel out residential care have lost the sense that what is in the best interest of the child is to have a home. Though thankfully rarely, sometimes that home is not a biological or foster family. I ask you to come to my case with an open mind.

References

Anglin, J. P., & Brendtro, L. K. (2017). Enduring wisdom: Towards a comprehensive history of professional child and youth care. *Scottish Journal of Residential Child Care, 16*. Retrieved from: https://www.celcis.org/application/files/7516/2308/2768/2017_Vol_16_3_Anglin_J_Enduring_wisdom.pdf.

Brown, W. K., & Seita, J. R. (Eds.). (2009). *Growing up in the care of strangers: The experiences, insights and recommendations of eleven former foster kids*. Tallahassee, FL: William Gladden Foundation Press.

Clough, R. (2005). Children in residence. In N. Axford, V. Berry, M. Little, & L. Morpeth (Eds.), *Forty years of research, policy and practice in children's services: A festschrift for Roger Bullock* (pp. 43–55). Oxford: Wiley-Blackwell.

Courtney, M. E., & Hughes-Heuring, D. (2009). Residential care in the United States of America: Past, present, and future. In M. E. Courtney & D. Iwaniec (Eds.), *Residential care of children: Comparative perspectives* (pp. 173–190). New York: Oxford Scholarship Online.

Doroshow, D. B. (2019). *Emotionally disturbed: A history of caring for America's troubled children.* Chicago, IL: University of Chicago Press.

English, P. C. (1984). Pediatrics and the unwanted child in history: Foundling homes, disease, and the origins of foster care in New York City, 1860 to 1920. *Pediatrics, 73*, 699–711. PMID: 6371697.

Flynn, J. R. (2016). *Does your family make you smarter?: Nature, nurture, and human autonomy.* Cambridge: Cambridge University Press.

Fulcher, L. C. (2009). Foreword. In M. Smith (Ed.), *Rethinking residential child care: Positive perspectives.* Bristol: Policy Press. doi: 10.1542/peds.97.4.569.

Geller, J. L. (2000). The last half-century of psychiatric services as reflected in *Psychiatric Services. Psychiatric Service, 51*, 41–67. doi: 10.1176/ps.51.1.41.

Gilligan, R. (2023). Residential care for children and youth in Ireland. In J. K. Whittaker, L. Holmes, J. F. del Valle, & S. James (Eds.), *Revitalizing residential care for children and youth: Cross-national trends and challenges* (pp. 108–122). Oxford: Oxford University Press. doi: 10.1093/oso/9780197644300.003.0008.

Goffman, E. (1961). *Asylums: Essays on the social situation of mental patients and other inmates.* Chicago, IL: Aldine Publishing.

Goldhaber, D. (2012). *The nature-nurture debates: Bridging the gap.* New York: Cambridge University Press.

Goldman, P. S., Bakermans-Kranenburg, M. J., Bradford, B., Christopoulos, A., Ken, P. L. A., Cuthbert, C., ... Sonuga-Barke, E. J. S. (2020). Institutionalisation and deinstitutionalisation of children 2: Policy and practice recommendations for global, national, and local actors. *Lancet Child and Adolescent Health, 4*, 606–633. doi: 10.1016/S2352-4642(20)30060-2.

Goode, D., Hill, D. B., Reiss, J., & Bronston, W. (2013). *A history and sociology of the Willowbrook State School.* Washington, DC: American Association on Intellectual and Developmental Disabilities.

Higginbotham, P. (2017). *Children's homes: A history of institutional care for Britain's young.* Barnsley: Pen & Sword History.

Jacobs, M. D. (2006). Indian boarding schools in comparative perspective: The removal of indigenous children in the United States and Australia, 1880-1940. In C. E. Trafzer, J. A. Keller, & L. Sisquoc (Eds.), *Boarding school blues: Revisiting American Indian educational experiences* (pp. 202–231). Lincoln: University of Nebraska Press.

Jones, M. B. (1993). Decline of the American orphanage, 1941-1980. *Social Services Review, 67*, 459–480. doi: 10.1086/603999.

King, L. S., Humphreys, K. L., & Gotlib, I. H. (2019). The neglect-enrichment continuum: Characterizing variation in early caregiving environments. *Developmental Review, 51*, 109–122. doi: 10.1016/j.dr.2019.01.001.

Knorth, E. J., & Harder, A. T. (2023). Residential care for children and youth in the Netherlands: High difficulties in low lands. In J. K. Whittaker, L. Holmes, J. F. del Valle, & S. James (Eds.), *Revitalizing residential care for children and youth: Cross-national trends and challenges* (pp. 193–208). Oxford: Oxford University Press. doi: 10.1093/oso/9780197644300.003.0014.

Lock, M., & Palsson, G. (2016). *Can science resolve the nature/nurture debate?* Cambridge: Cambridge University Press.

MacLean, K. (2003). The impact of institutionalization on child development. *Development and Psychopathology, 15*, 853–884. doi: 10.1017.S0954579403000415.

McKenzie, R. B. (Ed.). (2009). *Home away from home: The forgotten history of orphanages*. New York: Encounter Books.

Millham, S., Bullock, R., & Cherrett, P. (1975). *After grace, teeth: A comparative study of the residential experience of boys in approved schools*. London: Chaucer.

Proceedings of the Conference on the Care of Dependent Children. (1909). Washington, DC: Government Printing Office.

Rotabi, K. S., Roby, J. L., & Bunker, K. M. (2017). Altruistic exploitation: Orphan tourism and global social work. *British Journal of Social Work*, *47*, 648–665. doi: 10.1093/bjsw/bcv147.

Skeels, H. M. (1966). Adult status of children with contrasting early life experiences. *Monographs of the Society for Research in Child Development*, *31*(3), 1–65. doi: 10.2307/1165791.

Smith, E. P. (1995). Bring back the orphanages?: What policymakers of today can learn from the past. *Child Welfare*, *74*, 115–142. Retrieved from: https://www.proquest.com/scholarly-journals/bring-back-orphanages-what-policymakers-today-can/docview/213805999/se-2.

Smith, M. (2009). *Rethinking residential care: Positive perspectives*. Bristol: The Policy Press.

Stout, M. A. (2012). *Native American boarding schools*. Santa Barbara, CA: Greenwood.

Trent, J. W. (2016). *Inventing the feeble mind: A history of intellectual disability in the United States* (2nd ed.). New York: Oxford University Press.

Wang, L. K. (2016). *Outsourced children: Orphanage care and adoption in globalizing China*. Stanford, CA: Stanford University Press.

Whittaker, J. K., Holmes, L., del Valle, J. F., & James, S. (2023a). Future prospects and challenges for residential care for children and youth: Seeking direction from a cross-national analysis. In J. K. Whittaker, L. Holmes, J. F. del Valle, & S. James (Eds.), *Revitalizing residential care for children and youth: Cross-national trends and challenges* (pp. 429–442). New York: Oxford University Press. doi: 10.1093/oso/9780197644300.003.0029.

Whittaker, J. K., Holmes, L., del Valle, J. F., & James, S. (Eds.). (2023b). *Revitalizing residential care for children and youth: Cross-national trends and challenges*. New York: Oxford University Press.

Wolins, M. (Ed.). (1974). *Successful group care: Explorations in the powerful environment*. Chicago, IL: Aldine Publishing.

Woolford, A. (2015). *This benevolent experiment: Indigenous boarding school, genocide, and redress in Canada and the United States*. Lincoln: University of Nebraska Press.

2 Not a Good Place to Grow?

The two cases described in this chapter illustrate the issues surrounding residential care for children and youth that I address in the rest of the book.

A Senate Hearing: No Place to Grow Up

On May 19, 2015, the Committee on Finance of the United States Senate held a hearing, "No Place to Grow Up: How to Safely Reduce Reliance on Foster Care Group Homes" (*No place to grow up: How to safely reduce reliance on foster care group homes*, 2015). Many of the elements of this book are embodied in the testimony presented at the hearing and the communications provided in the hearing report. The hearing and report were part of the groundwork for the Family First Prevention Services Act (FFPSA) of 2018, amending Title IV-E of the Social Security Act, the passage of which eventually engendered my specific interest in the topic. The title of the hearing suggests it was organized with a particular conclusion in mind and the included testimony was clearly orchestrated to confirm the biases of most of the participants. However, much of the testimony helps define all sides of the issues.

One of the witnesses present before the committee was a 22-year-old woman named Lexie. Lexie related her experience with the child welfare system in Connecticut. Her removal from her biological family by child welfare, the reasons for which she did not want to describe, led to her placement with an uncle's family. Welfare workers soon after removed her from that home because, according to them, there were insufficient bedrooms in her uncle's house. Lexie testified that she was taken to an emergency shelter, then, over the next few weeks, to a series of foster care placements of various lengths, including one that lasted a single day. Eventually she was reunited with her family of origin, but when that did not work out, she was taken to a therapeutic group home. Lexie spent the next year and a half at the group home before leaving for college, a transition for which she felt ill-prepared. During college breaks, she had no place to go. Lexie described the group home as sterile, affectionless (affectionless by policy—touching by staff was considered a problem), oblivious to her trauma, and as a place where medications were used for control. The staff members operated in rotating shifts, and, by

DOI: 10.4324/9781003435709-2

Lexie's assessment, were overworked and underpaid. Their reason for being there was transactional, and that model, according to Lexie, led some of her fellow residents to engage in sex trafficking.

As part of the Senate hearing, Joo Yeun Chang, Associate Commissioner, Children's Bureau, Administration on Children, Youth, and Families, Department of Health and Human Services, representing the Obama administration's position, presented descriptive data indicating that being in a group home was correlated with factors such as having multiple emotional and behavioral problems, being older, having been previously adopted, and having had three or more previous placements. Based on these correlations, she said her office and the administration had made efforts to get states to decrease the use of what they called "congregate care." In her written testimony, Chang indicated that she had worked for the Casey Family Programs Foundation where they worked to get states to shift from placing children in congregate care to in-family programs such as therapeutic foster care and family reunification.

The private childcare sector was represented at the hearing by Jeremy Kohomban, President and CEO of The Children's Village in New York. Kohomban apologized for his organization's complicity in ineffective residential care as a regular method for dealing with children and youth. He stated that the evidence indicates children fare best in families, citing a "recent policy statement" about the importance of attachment from the American Psychological Association (APA). [Note: The statement Kohomban cited was not from the American Psychological Association. It was a statement from the American Orthopsychiatric Association whose journal is published by the APA. I have a detailed critique of this statement, Dozier et al., 2014, in Chapter 4.] Like others who testified, Kohomban argued for a limited role for residential care in providing short-term psychiatric care (a provision that was retained in the final version of the FFPSA of 2018). He suggested that private care providers change their business models, like his organization has done. He warned the senators:

> You may hear complaints from private providers in your district. They may say this kind of change is hard. Or that the needs of children and families cannot be met using these new models of care. *But the evidence is not on their side*. And we know that this kind of evolution is challenging to the tradition of "rescuing" children from their families and communities.
>
> (*No place to grow up: How to safely reduce reliance on foster care group homes*, 2015, p. 38, my emphasis)

The senators at the hearing were not there to hear new information. The hearing was a clear representation of the conventional wisdom. Two senators literally were not present but left written testimony. The testimony of those absentees and some who were there, along with the title of the hearing, indicate that they had made up their minds about group homes before the hearing. Senator Orrin Hatch, chairman of the committee wrote: "Group homes, sometimes referred to as 'congregate care,' are literally breeding grounds for the sexual exploitation of children and youth" (p. 32). He provided no evidence that that was true. Some senators saw more nuance. For example, Senator Ron Wyden was less definitively negative: "There's no question that residential care can play a crucial role in the foster care system" (p. 41). He also noted that all kinds of group homes were being lumped together: "The terms 'congregate care,' 'group homes' and 'residential treatment' are often used interchangeably; but the structure and quality of these settings varies widely as our witnesses will show" (p. 42). Other written testimony appended to the hearing transcript gave explicit recognition that there was good group care or that there was a place for group care in the child welfare system. Although the general tenor of the report fit its "no place to grow up" title, one communication, from the Alliance for Strong Families and Communities, cautioned that the hostility reflected in the hearing threatened the existence of residential care that is sorely needed for some children and youth: "...we are quite concerned by the rhetoric and policy proposals that paint residential as uniformly bad for children, or seek to make it difficult for systems to place children in residential settings" (p. 44).

They note that when residential care is used as a "last resort" because it is expensive, rather than when it could be most effective, the loser is the child.

Pages of Research Citations: Science Cancels Residential Care?

The FFPSA did not pass immediately following the 2015 Senate hearing. A few opponents, including a powerful North Carolina senator, were concerned that the act was taking funds away from a good, so-called "congregate care," to fund another good, "prevention services" ("robbing Peter to pay Paul,"). The Act's advocates did not give up. In February 2018 the Families First Prevention Service Act passed, essentially unchanged from the 2015 version (Lindell, Sorenson, & Mangold, 2020). The legislation has two major provisions (Lindell et al., 2020). The first is the laudable goal of trying to keep children and youth out of foster care. It allows federal funds to be used to provide a wide array of services to families, including drug and alcohol rehabilitation for parents, family counseling, and training in parenting skills. The second purpose is to reduce the use of group care for children and youth (although it allows the use of funds for youth over 18 for independent living group care). Except for very short-term exceptions (usually two weeks), federal funds are no longer to be used to provide a home to neglected or abused children in group care, even if they have a long history of failures in adoptive and/or family foster care.

Not long after passage of the bill, while states were trying to adapt their child welfare procedures to accommodate the provisions of the act, the *Carolina Public Press* (July 9, 2018) published an article by Michael

Gebelein about the concerns children's homes in North Carolina had about the consequences for children, youth and homes from the passing of the act (https://carolinapublicpress.org/28028/future-uncertain-for-thousands-of-nc-children-in-group-homes/). Among others, I was quoted as Chair of the Board of Directors at North Carolina's Black Mountain Home for Children, Youth and Families (along with the Home's president): "For some children and youth, family-style residential care like we provide is the best environment for their situation." Many of the children the Home supports in their residential component (like many modern American children's homes, Black Mountain also has emergency foster care, foster care, and transitional, and independent living components as part of its array of services) have been in many previous family foster care homes (sometimes 20 or 30 or more before the age of 15) or are in sibling groups larger than almost any family foster care provider could (or should) serve. Many other similar children's homes were in the same position.

Immediately after publication of the *Carolina Public Press* article, Richard Wexler, on letterhead that indicated that he was Executive Director of the National Coalition for Child Protection Reform in Alexandria Virginia, posted a response to the *Carolina Public Press* article (Wexler, 2018). Mr. Wexler is a journalist/family advocate who is against residential care in any form. He claims he can provide a long list of news articles on residential care settings gone wrong (he is less interested in adoptive, foster, or biological families that have gone wrong). In his post, Wexler claimed that reporter Gebelein should have focused on the "*enormous harm*" (my emphasis) done by "institutions" ("latter-day orphanages") described in the article. In a list of contentious "In fact" bullets, it is Wexler's first that concerns us here (emphasis is mine):

In fact:

- The *evidence is overwhelming* that group homes and other institutions harm children. It takes *three single-spaced pages just to list the citations on the research*. And it doesn't matter how pretty they are or how gooey the rhetoric is on their websites. What the head of one institution calls "family-style residential care," is an oxymoron.

Reading this presented me with a personal dilemma. Wexler tells me that research and scholarship show that residential care is an unequivocal evil. My doctoral training at a prestigious research institution (the University of Minnesota's Institute of Child Development) biased me to accept good scholarship. However, my experience with residential care was inconsistent with the notion that residential care is an unequivocal evil. Should I trust the research or what I had witnessed? Wexler kindly made his three pages of research evidence available in his response (Wexler, 2018). The citation list gave me an opportunity to consider his evidence, all three pages, that residential care should be eliminated. I was off to the library.

Here is what I found after sorting through, best I could, the list, negotiating multiple citation errors among the 40 items (the undated "literature review" is credited to Richard A. Wayman, J.D. who was, at the time of the review, associated with an agency helping homeless youth in Minnesota). Bear with me. Evaluating the research base behind the hostility toward residential care is central to my case. Wexler represents the conventional wisdom.

Inaccessible or irrelevant sources. First, I could not access three of the cited sources. One (Roy) is an unpublished 1983 paper titled "Is continuity enough?: Substitute care and socialization." However, Michael Rutter, a prominent researcher in developmental psychology, refers to Roy's paper in one of his published chapters. He summarized the findings as indicating that children from institutions show numerous deficits. The institutions and the children involved are not described. The contents of Rutter (1981), and a chapter by Triseliotis and Hill (1990) are cited in some of the literature covered in Chapters 4 and 5 (in other work Triseliotis provides interesting qualitative, retrospective data, especially on adoption and fostering, and argues for adoption because of the security it provides the child, e.g., Triseliotis, 2002). References to those sources do not support the idea of "enormous harm" from residential care (see the recent comment by Rutter and his colleagues at the end of the section on infants, below).

Another six of the sources in Wexler's three pages seem to have been included in error. The empirical aspect of Berry's (1975) book reports the results from questionnaires given to 44 social work students in Britain. Its main point is that childcare workers should serve an apprenticeship with a skilled mentor. The reference listed as being authored by a K. Josh in *CQ Quarterly* is apparently a piece by Kenneth Jost, a Washington lawyer and journalist, in *CQ Researcher* (Jost, 1991). Jost's article focuses on the American foster care crisis of the 1980s. It mentions orphanages in historical context and briefly mentions the debate surrounding the possible role of "new" orphanages in solving the foster care crisis of that period. The Olds and Henderson (1989) chapter's inclusion among the sources also must be an error. It reports a study of the effect of home visits by nurses on instances of abuse. It does not address the effects of residential care on children in any way. Zoccolillo, Pickles, Quinton, and Rutter's (1992) paper focuses on adults who had been in group-cottage children's homes at one time, but the relevance of this paper to the question of the effects of residential care is not apparent. Sroufe (1991) is a six-paragraph item in a non-refereed newsletter that attempts to distinguish bonding and attachment. It says nothing about residential care. The Reinhard (1985) citation is to a brief theoretical article in German about coping, loss, and child psychopathology (it is indexed in the Web of Science with a different title translation than that given in Wexler's list). It provides no data on the harm caused by residential care.

Opinion pieces or histories. Seven of the 40 sources are opinion pieces or histories. One of them (Aring, 1991) is a *defense* of "orphanages." Three are opinion pieces about the unserious mid-1990s debate initiated by conservative

American Republican politicians about using orphanages as an aid in solving the American welfare problem (Frank, Kass, Earls, & Eisenberg, 1996; Markel, 1995; Smith, 1995). That debate died out when it became clear that the proposal was neither fiscally nor ethically justifiable. The other three sources are about the history of group care, one about 18th century care (Radbill, 1976), one *laudatory* history of a New York City orphanage that closed in 1941 (Bogen, 1992), and a history of care in New York City from 1860 to 1920 (English, 1984). None of these papers provide evidence that 21st century residential care causes "enormous harm" to children.

Research on infants in institutions. The largest group of sources in Wexler's three pages includes 14 articles about the effects of institutionalization of infants in group settings (varying from hospitals to old-style orphanages) on infant development. There are seven classic articles on pre-1960 institutions or hospital settings with large infant to caretaker ratios in the United States or Britain. It was research like this that led to the closing of the few settings that still offered institutional care to infants in mid-20th century America and the United Kingdom. Bowlby's (1951) report summarizes much of the research in the older papers in this list and adds his own reflections from the plight of children separated from their parents during the Second World War. Brennemann (1932) writes about the infant wards of hospitals of a century ago and the high mortality involved when children with serious diseases were treated together in the horrific conditions in large hospital wards. Chapin's (1915) historic editorial position (a sensible one indeed) is that sick infants and "foundlings and abandoned babies" need individualized care. The Goldfarb (1945) paper is just one of a series of articles by Goldfarb reporting on his longitudinal study of infants from an institution operating during the 1930s. Goldfarb, comparing institutionalized children to children who had experienced dysfunctional parenting, found that the effects of institutionalization during infancy had their most profound influences in the development of abstract thinking.

Provence and Lipton's (1962) *Infants in institutions* does not meet modern standards of research in terms of design and measurement. Regardless, it makes a convincing case that stark differences in environment do matter. Infants should receive personalized care in their first year. A couple of decades later, however, Provence argued that stable institutions might be better than the enormous number of placements some infants experience in foster care (Provence, 1989 as cited in McCall, 1999). Skeels' (1966) paper is a follow-up of the famous 1930s' Iowa Child Welfare study of "experimental" infants who got more attention from "mother-surrogates" (women at another institution for individuals with mental disabilities). Eleven of 13 experimental infants were subsequently adopted. None of the "contrast group" of 12 were adopted. The later life experiences of those who were adopted and stimulated were much more positive. Although the original 1930s' study has a place in my heart (several of the original investigators are among my intellectual grandparents), the study has received devastating criticism going back to 1940. Even those of us who firmly believe that intelligence can be modified in stimulating environments long ago stopped citing this line of research except in the history of psychology course. Spitz's (1965) book was originally published in French in 1954. One of the institutions in which the infants were studied was described as "bleak" and the other was a penal institution to which pregnant, "delinquent" girls were committed. Spitz's work is clouded by an outmoded theory of psychological development and methodological issues, but anyone who has seen his films would attest that neither of these institutions was good for the infants (I watched one in the very first class of my first child psychology course in 1969 and was appalled indeed).

Four of the 14 sources on infants Wexler points us to are from Tizard's longitudinal study of the same set of 65 children who entered residential nurseries in Britain before the age of four months (Tizard & Joseph, 1970; Tizard & Rees, 1975). By age 4½ years, 24 had been adopted, 15 had been restored to their family of origin, and 26 had remained in institutional care. Tizard and Hodges (1978) report on the children's status at age eight years when eight of the children were still in an institution. The children who remained in institutions over a long period had experienced many different caretakers. The results from these studies are complicated and selection factors and the small size of the groups make conclusions difficult. However, it is clear that those children who had been adopted were doing the best by age 4½ and by eight years. They had the highest IQs and fewest behavior problems. However, at 4½ years, the institutionalized group displayed no more behavior problems than a comparison group of London home-reared children of the same age. The conclusions of the 1978 paper include that the children still in the institution "were not retarded" (p. 117) and that the adopted group "had the highest mean I.Q. and reading achievement; this finding appears to be related to the higher social class of the adoptive parents and the poorer emotional adjustment of the children restored to their biological families" (p. 117). In the final paper on the longitudinal study, Hodges and Tizard (1989) are strongest in their indictment of the effects of early institutional care (social, not cognitive), but the last follow-up included only seven restored children and 14 adopted children. The authors suggest that multiple caregivers and the lack of the development of a secure attachment in the first two years were the likely factors in the children's developmental problems.

The final three sources related to infants in the list do not seem to belong. Collard (1971) studied exploratory and play behaviors of infants reared in an institution and in lower- and middle-class homes. Although this paper is plagued by methodological problems (of measurement and sample selection), this simple study shows that 16 infants of mixed ethnicity in institutions explored less than white working- and upper-middle-class infants. Rheingold's (spelled Reingold in the list) dissertation at the University of Chicago (Rheingold, 1956) says nothing about "enormous harm" done by institutions. It simply shows that infant social behavior could be modified by decreasing the number of caregivers that an infant encounters. Hunt, Mohandessi, Ghodssi and Akiyama (1976) did study five "waves" of children in an Iranian orphanage who were tested on an infant development instrument. Waves in which there was systematic stimulation did better than waves that did not. The fifth wave of 11 infants did the best, surpassing norms from infants of professional families in America. It is hard to see the relevance of this study to Wexler's argument.

Although mostly very old, the relevant sources in Wexler's list on infants suggest a sensible conclusion that infants need as close to 1 on 1 care as is practicable. It is curious that there are no references in the list, provided to the general public in 2018 (and still available in 2023), to the much more recent research literature in high-quality journals on the short-term or long-term effects of the infamous and horrific Romanian orphanages on infants (the Frank et al. paper above does). I know no one in modern childcare who would advocate anything but parental (natural or foster) care for infants and toddlers except in extreme emergencies for short periods. I will simply reiterate that no one in professional care that I know of is advocating for any kind of group care for infants and toddlers under any normal circumstances. Moreover, no licensed "institution" in a developed country that I know of resembles the Romanian "orphanages," Czech "baby institutes," Iranian or Iowan orphanages, hospital wards, or any of the other institutional settings for infants from the past as characterized in these articles. Unfortunately, it is probably this very literature that is most responsible for creating the stereotype of the "orphanage" or "institution," the conventional wisdom, that is still being applied to residential childcare today by people like Mr. Wexler.

Interestingly, because so many infants are separated from their parents in very poor countries where finding family care for infants is difficult, some researchers have taken a new look at early institutional care. For instance, a recent article co-authored by the late Michael Rutter, the co-author of several items in Wexler's list, concludes:

> Thus, much of the literature seeks to conclude that early institutional rearing is inevitably damaging. *The evidence does not support that.* Rather, it suggests that it is a risk factor but the most profound effects are seen only *when the rearing is accompanied by gross deprivation,* as it was in the Romanian sample.
>
> (Woodhouse, Miah, & Rutter, 2018, p. 8, my emphases)

Moreover, The St. Petersburg-USA Orphanage Research Team (2008) offers evidence that the development of infants and young children in Russian "baby homes" can be enhanced by reducing child-caregiver ratios, providing more consistency in caregivers, and training caregivers to be more sensitive and responsive in their interactions with children.

Potentially relevant sources. What remains of the 40 references are ten sources in Wexler's list that could be relevant to a conclusion that residential care for children and youth (the kind he was specifically attacking) is enormously harmful. I will take them in chronological order of publication.

Tizard, Cooperman, Joseph, and Tizard (1972) is more focused than Tizard's studies of infant institutionalization. The children in this study were three- to five-year-olds in residential care (the three facilities involved were associated with Dr. Barnardo's Society, the Church of England Children's Society, and the National Children's Home). The focus of the study was the relationship of adult talk directed at children and indicators of their language development. "No "institutional retardation" was found, and the mean test scores on both verbal and nonverbal tests were average" (abstract, p. 337). The authors conclude that their evidence

> strongly suggests that intellectual retardation is not a necessary consequence of institutional placement; even in our "worst" nurseries the mean test scores were all average, while in the "best" nurseries the children's language scores were considerably above average. Since many of the children were of lower-working-class parentage, it seems likely that intellectually they had in fact benefited from their institutional upbring.
>
> (pp. 355–356)

Obviously, this study does not support Wexler's position.

Wolkind's (1974) study of school-age children (ages five to 12 years) who had been in a "large children's home" for at least six months is descriptive. The author concludes that so-called "affectionless psychopathy disorder" and the time in care are "secondary to the family situation" (p. 219, emphasis in original). Furthermore,

> ...the results of the study indicate that to attempt at all costs to keep a child with its own family would not be the way to prevent the development of psychiatric disorders. Many of the children appear to be severely damaged by their experiences prior to the admission.
>
> (p. 219)

Again, this study does not support Mr. Wexler's position.

The research summarized in Langmeier and Matejcek's (1975) book is from the 1950s and before. It summarizes research on extreme deprivation from animal studies (e.g., Harlow's studies of wire and cloth monkey mothers, Harlow, 1958), case studies (e.g., Victor, the wild boy of Aveyron who apparently grew up in the wild during the late 18th and early 19th centuries, Itard, 1962), and mortality data from 18th and 19th century foundling homes. The most relevant original research reported here involves Czech "baby institutes" (as asserted above, group care is not for infants) and of children who had experienced group care in their preschool years. The group care is not well-described, but pictures in the book suggest high child to adult ratios. The focus of the researchers is on what they consider to be "cultural" deprivation and the need to use group care only in serious cases of family dysfunction. Bush's (1980) data are retrospective reports by 370 children in 1975. The sampling technique is first described as random, then as stratified. Of the 370 children, 269 had lived in one of 100 different institutions at some point. At the time of the study 51 were in 17 different institutions and 39 in 17 different group homes. Neither the institutions nor the group homes are described. A survey of unestablished reliability and validity was used on this odd sample and results are reported for foster homes, group homes, institutions, relatives' homes, independent living or living with natural parents. Unfortunately, the data analytic strategy used violates all kinds of procedural safeguards (e.g., ad hoc tests and multiple comparisons without controls, analysis of single-item measures of unknowable reliability, and unreported effect sizes). Regardless, the author concludes that institutions were rated worst by the children and group homes share some of the problems of institutions. However, the author's own data show on several items (Table 1, Bush, 1980, p. 243) that group homes were rated as better places to live than living with natural parents. The author also conceded that the institutions represented in the sample did not include the "top-ranked sites" in 1975.

Rindfleisch and Rabb (1984) ask: How much of a problem is resident mistreatment in child welfare institutions? Unfortunately, they relied on voluntarily returned questionnaires to obtain their data from 1,700 institutions. For 1980, they reported 119 confirmed complaints at residential institutions. Despite definitional/standard sensitivity differences between kinds of care, in short, the answer to the authors' question was "too high." They comment that "The data seem to us to confirm the possibility that harm to residents can occur in a field in which many facilities are doing an excellent job" (p. 40). This issue is treated better in Shealy's article, below. The Quinton, Rutter and Liddle (1984) and Rutter and Quinton (1984) sources report a retrospective study of two groups of women first studied in the 1960s. Ninety-four had been institutionalized because of parenting problems. A comparison group of 51 were from the general population. In the first article, at ages 21–27 years, the women who had been institutionalized showed lower levels of psychosocial functioning, and more problems in their own parenting. Unsurprisingly, these deficits were significantly ameliorated among women who had a non-deviant spouse and good living conditions. The second report, with some minor differences, is the same report as in the previous paper (it is on the same group of formerly institutionalized women, but ten of the comparison group have disappeared). Women who had been institutionalized were doing much worse in young adulthood "except for a sizable minority." The women in that group were currently in good psychosocial situations. These studies were apparently the beginning of Rutter's interest in resiliency, a topic he has written about extensively since.

Most of the analyses in Colton (1988) are "sociological," by which the author appears to mean "qualitative." The programs compared were "special foster homes" (described as homes for children too old for traditional foster home placement) and "Children's Homes." Colton's conclusion is that the foster homes seemed to be more child-oriented but that data from the children were not different enough to make firm conclusions. He notes that the Children's Homes were greatly improved over those of the 1940s and that there was ... "grounds for optimism rather than gloom" ... (p. 41) in regard to the institutions. Gomez, Sos, Randall, and Vaquero (1991) studied the social integration strategies of five four- to five-year-olds reared in an institution compared to those of seven home-reared children. The authors report that there were some differences in the strategies the two groups used but that no causal relationship with institutionalization could be inferred.

Finally, Shealy (1995—in Wexler's list it is listed as appearing in *Arch Pediatr Adolesc Med.*, but it clearly was published in *American Psychologist*) does not provide any new data. Instead, his is a nuanced piece that concludes that out-of-home care is not necessarily bad or good. The quality of the care is what is crucial (we will return to this issue throughout this book). Shealy goes a long way toward outlining what quality care is. He also neatly dispels the many myths about welfare families that were common during the mid-1990s debates about welfare reform and that are still so prevalent today. Shealy does not support the notion from the American right political wing that the early 20th century orphanages should be reestablished. But he also says "...home removal is always preferable to an abusive, neglectful, or emotionally damaging environment that is unsafe or cannot be modified with skillful intervention" (Shealy, 1995, p. 574).

Summary. What can we make of Wexler's "three single-spaced pages just to list the citations on the research"? Nine of the 40 references are inaccessible or irrelevant, seven are opinion pieces or histories, 14 are on infants reared in deprived environments (although three of those appear to have been included in error). Only ten of the cited works are at all relevant to care for children and youth, the kind of care Wexler is criticizing. This body of research Wexler pointed us to in 2018 is badly outdated and highly selective. None of it was published in this century. The types of "institutions" involved no longer exist in North America or Western Europe, and, in most cases, have not existed for a long time. The research leaves out much recent work that provides more nuanced and optimistic views of residential care (e.g., Farmer, Murray, Ballentine, Rauktis, & Burns, 2017; Farmer, Seifert, Wagner, Burns, & Murray, 2017; McKenzie, 1997, 2003; Thompson, Smith, Osgood, Dowd, Friman, & Daly, 1996; Whetten et al., 2011). The studies included suffer from numerous methodological problems. Almost none of the studies would meet modern standards for peer reviewed publishable research.

Even if we take the research in Wexler's list at face value, there is no convincing evidence that the residential care provided by the wide variety of programs cause "enormous harm" to children. *The cited literature in the list he gives us simply does not say what Wexler says it does.* The citations reviewed above on infants are also outdated, but there is more recent research that we will examine in Chapter 4.

The Bigger Picture

The 2015 Senate committee hearing and Wexler's response to a 2018 news article serve to illustrate several central themes in the rest of this book. First, the hostile nature of the rhetoric about residential care is evident. Second, there is a lack of clarity in lumping widely differing forms of residential care together. The terms "institution," "congregate care," and "group home" are especially problematic (Chow, Mettrick, Stephan, & Von Waldner, 2014). They are applied to organizations that provide family-style homes with sophisticated programming and 24-7 staff on weekly shifts, to isolated houses staffed by poorly paid and trained staff on shifts, and to institutions around the world that simply warehouse infants and young children. The pejorative terms "congregate" and "institution" conjure up visions of barracks-like dormitories, massive food halls, and large child-to-caregiver ratios that are not consistent with modern quality residential care. They are terms rarely used by advocates of high-quality residential care. The lumping of very different experiences makes much of the residential care research difficult to interpret. Third, discussions of residential care frequently suffer from reliance on anecdotes or assertions not supported by research evidence. The most compelling testimony in the Senate hearing came from Lexie. But how representative is her experience? What happened to Lexie and others should not have happened. Again, the real issue is the quality of care that children and youth receive. Finally, the Senate hearing illustrates the frequent overgeneralization of the limited research on residential care across settings, age groups, and countries. Many writers are facile in their generalization of infant research to older children and youth in very different residences. Legislators, foundation directors, and even research scholars have been guilty. The residential care literature is replete with "we know," "research shows," and "experts say" statements that are simply not accurate. It is important to apply research tools in evaluating the residential care literature. The next chapter provides a brief overview of those tools.

References

Aring, C. D. (1991). In defense of orphanages. *American Scholar*, *60*, 575–579.
Berry, J. (1975). *Daily experience in residential life: A study of children and their care-givers*. London: Routledge & Kegan Paul.

Bogen, H. (1992). *The luckiest orphans: A history of the Hebrew Orphan Asylum of New York*. Urbana: University of Illinois Press.
Bowlby, J. (1951). *Maternal care and mental health*. Geneva: World Health Organization. Monograph No. 2.
Brennemann, J. (1932). The infant ward. *American Journal of the Diseases of Children, 43*, 577–584. doi: 10.1001/archpedi.1932.01950030047007.
Bush, M. (1980). Institutions for dependent and neglected children: Therapeutic option of choice or last resort? *American Journal of Orthopsychiatry, 50*, 239–255. doi: 10.1111/j.1939-0025.1980.tb03287.x.
Chapin, H. D. (1915). Are institutions necessary for infants? *Journal of the American Medical Association, 65*, 1–3. doi: 10.1001/jama.1915.02570270003001.
Chow, W.-Y., Mettrick, J. E., Stephan, S. H., & Von Waldner, C. A. (2014). Youth in group home care: Youth characteristics and predictors of later functioning. *Journal of Behavioral Health Services & Research, 41*, 503–519. doi: 10.1007/s11414-012-9282-2.
Collard, R. R. (1971). Exploratory and play behaviors of infants reared in an institution and in lower- and middle-class homes. *Child Development, 42*, 1003–1015. doi: 10.2307/1127787.
Colton, M. (1988). Foster and residential care practices compared. *British Journal of Social Work, 18*, 25–42. doi: 10.2307/1127787.
Dozier, M., Kaufman, J., Kobak, R., O'Connor, T. G., Sagi-Schwartz, A., Scott, S., ... Zeanah, C. H. (2014). Consensus statement on group care for children and adolescents: A statement of Policy of the American Orthopsychiatric Association. *American Journal of Orthopsychiatry, 84*, 219–225. doi: 10.1037/ort0000005.
English, P. C. (1984). Pediatrics and the unwanted child in history: Foundling homes, disease, and the origins of foster care in New York City, 1860 to 1920. *Pediatrics, 73*, 699–711. PMID: 6371697.
Farmer, E. M. Z., Murray, M., Ballentine, K., Rauktis, M. E., & Burns, B. J. (2017). Would we know it if we saw it?: Assessing quality of care in group homes for youth. *Journal of Emotional and Behavioral Disorders, 25*, 28–36. doi: 10.1177/1063426616687363
Farmer, E. M. Z., Seifert, H., Wagner, H. R., Burns, B. J., & Murray, M. (2017). Does model matter?: Examining change across time for youth in group homes. *Journal of Emotional and Behavioral Disorders, 25*, 119–128. doi: 10.1177/1063426616630520.
Frank, D. A., Klass, P. E., Earls, F., & Eisenberg, L. (1996). Infants and young children in orphanages: One view from pediatrics and child psychiatry. *Pediatrics, 97*, 569–578. doi: 10.1542/peds.97.4.569.
Goldfarb, W. (1945). Psychological privation in infancy and subsequent adjustment. *American Journal of Orthopsychiatry, 15*, 247–255. doi: 10.1111/j.1939-0025.1945.tb04938.x.
Gomez, C., Sos, F., Randall, C., & Vaquero, E. (1991). Estudio comparado del comportamiento de niños educados en medio familiar y niños educados en instituciones. Una perspectiva etológica. [A comparative study of behavior of children reared at home and children reared in institutions: An ethnological perspective.] *Infancia y Aprendizaje, 56*, 105–122.
Harlow, H. F. (1958). The nature of love. *American Psychologist, 13*, 673–685. doi: 10.1037/h0047884.

Hodges, J., & Tizard, B. (1989). IQ and behavioural adjustment of ex-institutional adolescents. *Journal of Child Psychology and Psychiatry*, *30*, 53–75. doi: 10.1111/j.1469-7610.1989.tb00769.x.

Hunt, J. M., Mohandessi, K., Ghodssi, M., & Akiyama, M. (1976). The psychological development of orphanage-reared infants: Interventions with outcomes (Tehran). *Genetic Psychology Monographs*, *94*, 177–226. PMID: 992359.

Itard, J.-M. G. (1962). *The wild boy of Aveyron*. New York: Appleton-Century-Crofts.

Jost, K. (1991, September 27). Foster care crisis. *CQ Researcher*, *1*, 705–278. http://library.cqpress.com/

Langmeier, J., & Matejcek, Z. (1975). *Psychological deprivation in childhood* (original 1963 Czechoslovakian edition edited by G. L. Mangan). New York: Wiley.

Lindell, K. U., Sorenson, C. K., & Mangold, S. V. (2020). The Family First Prevention Services Act: A new era of child welfare reform. *Public Health Reports*, *135*, 282–286. doi: 10.1177/0033354919900892.

Markel, H. (1995). Orphanages revisited: Some historical perspectives on dependent, abandoned, and orphaned children in America. *Archives of Pediatrics and Adolescent Medicine*, *149*, 609–610. doi: 10.1001/archpedi.1995.02170190019002.

McCall, J. N. (1999). Research on the psychological effects of orphanage care: A critical review. In R. B. McKenzie (Ed.), *Rethinking orphanages in the 21st century* (127–150). Thousand Oaks, CA: Sage.

McKenzie, R. (1997). Orphanage alumni: How they have done and how they evaluate their experience. *Child & Youth Care Forum*, *26*, 87–111. doi: 10.1007/BF02589359.

McKenzie, R. B. (2003). The impact of orphanages on the alumni's lives and assessments of their childhoods. *Children and Youth Services Review*, *25*, 703–753. doi: 10.1016/S0190-7409(03)00068-9.

No place to grow up: How to safely reduce reliance on foster care group homes. Hearing before the Committee on Finance of the United States Senate (S. Hrg. 114–273), 114th Congress, May 19, 2015. Retrieved from: https://www.finance.senate.gov/imo/media/doc/20209.pdf.

Olds, D. L., & Henderson, C. R. (1989). The prevention of maltreatment. In D. Cicchetti & V. Carlson (Eds.), *Child Maltreatment: Theory and research on the consequences of child abuse and neglect* (pp. 722–763). Cambridge: Cambridge University Press.

Provence, S., & Lipton, R. C. (1962). *Infants in institutions: A comparison of their development with family-reared infants during the first year of life*. New York: International Universities Press.

Quinton, D., Rutter, M., & Liddle, C. (1984). Institutional rearing, parenting difficulties and marital support. *Psychological Medicine*, *14*, 107–124. doi: 10.1017/s0033291700003111.

Radbill, S. X. (1976). Reared in adversity: Institutional care of children in the 18th century. *American Journal of the Diseases of Children*, *130*, 751–761. doi: 10.1001/archpedi.1976.02120080073008.

Reinhard, H. G. (1985). Adjustment and personal loss. A contribution to the psychopathology of childhood and adolescence. *Nervenarzt*, *56*, 252–258. PMID: 4010828.

Rheingold, H. L. (1956). The modification of social responsiveness in institutional babies. *Monographs of the Society for Research in Child Development*, *21*(2), 1–48. doi: 10.2307/1165614.

Rindfleisch, N., & Rabb, J. (1984). How much of a problem is resident mistreatment in child welfare institutions? *Child Abuse & Neglect*, *8*, 33–40. doi: 10.1016/0145-2134(84)90047-4.

Rutter, M. (1981). *Maternal deprivation reassessed* (2nd ed.). New York: Penguin.

Rutter, M., & Quinton, D. (1984). Long-term follow-up of women institutionalized in childhood: Factors promoting good functioning in adult life. *British Journal of Developmental Psychology*, *2*, 191–204. doi: 10.1111/j.2044-835X.1984.tb00925.x.

Shealy, C. N. (1995). From *Boys Town* to *Oliver Twist*: Separating fact from fiction in welfare reform and out-of-home placement of children and youth. *American Psychologist*, *50*, 565–580. doi: 10.1037/0003-066X.50.8.565.

Skeels, H. M. (1966). Adult status of children with contrasting early life experiences. *Monographs of the Society for Research in Child Development*, *31*(3), 1–65. doi: 10.2307/1165791.

Smith, E. P. (1995). Bring back the orphanages?: What policymakers of today can learn from the past. *Child Welfare*, *74*, 115–142. Retrieved from: https://www.proquest.com/scholarly-journals/bring-back-orphanages-what-policymakers-today-can/docview/213805999/sc-2.

Spitz, R. A. (1965). *The first year of life: A psychoanalytic study of normal and deviant development of object relations*. New York: International Universities Press.

Sroufe, A. (1991). Sorting it out: Attachment and bonding. *Early Report: Center for Early Education and Development* (University of Minnesota), *18*(2), 3–4.

The St. Petersburg-USA Orphanage Research Team. (2008). The effects of early social-emotional and relationship experience on the development of young orphanage children. *Monographs of the Society for Research in Child Development*, *73*(3). doi: 10.1002/9781444309683.

Thompson, R. W., Smith, G. L., Osgood, D. W., Dowd, T. P., Friman, G. L., & Daly, D. L. (1996). Residential care: A study of short- long-term educational effects. *Children and Youth Services Review*, *18*, 221–242. doi: 10.1016/0190-7409(96)00002-3.

Tizard, B., Cooperman, O., Joseph, A., & Tizard, J. (1972). Environmental effects on language development: A study of young children in long-stay residential nurseries. *Child Development*, *43*, 337–358. doi: 10.2307/1127540.

Tizard, B., & Hodges, J. (1978). The effect of early institutional rearing on the development of eight year old children. *Journal of Child Psychology and Psychiatry*, *19*, 99–118. doi: 10.1111/j.1469-7610.1978.tb00453.x.

Tizard, B., & Joseph, A. (1970). Cognitive development of young children in residential care: A study of children aged 24 months. *Journal of Child Psychology and Psychiatry*, *11*, 177–186. doi: 10.1111/j.1469-7610.1970.tb01024.x.

Tizard, B., & Rees, J. (1975). The effect of early institutional rearing on the behaviour problems and affectional relationships of four-year-old children. *Journal of Child Psychology and Psychiatry*, *16*, 61–73. doi: 10.1111/j.1469-7610.1975.tb01872.x.

Triseliotis, J. (2002). Long-term foster care or adoption? The evidence examined. *Child and Family Social Work*, *7*, 23–33. doi: 10.1046/j.1365-2206.2002.00224.x.

Triseliotis, J., & Hill, M. (1990). Contrasting adoption, foster care and residential care. In D. M. Brodzinsky & M. D. Schechter (Eds.), *The psychology of adoption* (pp. 107–120). New York: Oxford University Press.

Wang, L. K. (2016). *Outsourced children: Orphanage care and adoption in globalizing China*. Stanford CA: Stanford University Press.

Wexler, R. (2018). *A response to the Carolina Public Press article about the Family First Act and "group homes."* Retrieved from: https://drive.google.com/file/d/1h8t8JKtrgHNFra8giP7M2Z41qL1Cfogs/view.

Whetten, K., Ostermann, J., Whetten, R., O'Donnell, K., Thielman, N., & Positive Outcomes for Orphans Team. (2011). More than the loss of a parent: Potentially traumatic events among orphaned and abandoned children. *Journal of Traumatic Stress*, *24*, 174–182. doi: 10.1002/jts.20625.

Woodhouse, S., Miah, A., & Rutter, M. (2018). A new look at the supposed risks of early institutional rearing. *Psychological Medicine*, *48*, 1–10. doi:10.1017/S0033291717001507

Wolkind, S. N. (1974). The components of "affectionless psychopathy" in institutionalized children. *Journal of Child Psychology and Psychiatry*, *15*, 215–220. doi: 10.1111/j.1469-7610.1974.tb01246.x.

Zoccolillo, M., Pickles, A., Quinton, D., & Rutter, M. (1992). The outcome of childhood conduct disorder: Implications for defining adult personality disorder and conduct disorder. *Psychological Medicine*, *22*, 971–986. doi: 10.1017/s003329170003854x

3 Reading the Residential Care Research Literature

Reading the literature on residential care presents numerous challenges. Much of the literature is plagued by imprecise language, insufficient descriptions, and overgenerous use of acronyms (I counted 17 acronyms in the 16 pages of a recent article). Moreover, doing good research in the real world is much more difficult than doing it under the controlled conditions of a laboratory. Measuring the complex constructs related to human behavior, personality, and intelligence is challenging. There are conceptual issues related to choosing the phenomena to be studied. There are ethical issues that limit what researchers can do. Designing experiments that allow for valid inferences requires adaptation and compromise. Sometimes things are so complex that making valid cause-effect inferences is impossible. Because of these complexities, I do not want to be overly critical. However, there are limits on what we can know and say from the kinds of research available, yet policymakers have made inappropriate inferences from limited data. Invalid inferences can have great consequences for children and families.

Residential care researchers frequently recognize the methodological difficulties I will discuss here. They mention them in the ubiquitous "limitations" sections of their articles. That recognition too often has not stopped them from applying conclusions to children and youth unlike those who were studied. It has not stopped them from making broad policy statements or including words like "effect" in the titles of their papers or in their conclusions when no cause-effect inferences are warranted.

The Components of a Research Study: Overview

The basic research methods are typically couched in terms of the "scientific method." Many researchers (and teachers of research methodology) consider *the* scientific method a useful myth (e.g., Bauer, 1992). There is no one infallible way of doing science. The philosophy of science I am most comfortable with is one that sees science as problem solving (Laudan, 1977). The job of the researcher is not to prove or disprove theories or hypotheses, to confirm hypotheses, to conform with a paradigm, or to find the Truth with a capital "T." It is to provide reasonable answers (or theoretical responses with a small "t")

DOI: 10.4324/9781003435709-3

to interesting questions. Better theories solve more problems and do it at a faster rate than competing theories. The basic components of the mythical scientific method most of us learned in school are useful tools, but those tools need to be used judiciously.

The first step in the elementary version of the so-called scientific method is the generation of a research question (or in more formal versions, a hypothesis) based on observation of anomalies, previous research, and/or a theory. In residential care research, there are interesting, although vague, questions such as "is residential care good for children and youth?" or "is type A care more effective than type B care?" Researchers may simply want to carefully describe a situation (**descriptive studies**). Or researchers want to make inferences about how one variable is related to or predicts another variable (**correlational studies**). If the question the researchers are addressing is one where the hypothesis is that one variable or treatment with multiple conditions (the independent variable, in residential care research, a type of care, intervention, treatment or therapy) causes or influences another variable (the dependent variable, "dependent" because its value depends on the independent variable), a scheme for relating the factors, called an **experimental or quasi-experimental research design,** is required. In descriptive, correlational, and experimental research, something gets measured (in experimental research it is the dependent variable). Relevant measurement instruments are taken off the shelf or newly developed to assess the relevant phenomena. In the area of residential care, these may be measures of behavioral, psychological, or educational constructs or outcomes like return to family of origin, adoption, permanent foster placement, years of education completed, or employment status. Finally, data are collected and analyzed and discussed in response to the hypothesis or question. Inevitably, the final point of discussion is that more research is needed. The rest of this chapter will focus on the major steps in more detail.

The Uses of Theory in the Residential Care Research: Research Questions

If the research process frequently begins with a theory, can we identify a theory of residential care? In subsequent chapters we will encounter references to a variety of child development theories. They include attachment theory, peer contagion theory, operant conditioning theory, Anglin's pain theory, and Bronfenbrenner's ecological theory. Each has been used to explain why residential care might be harmful or helpful for children of a certain age. However, the simplistic contrast at a global level of "institutional" (group, congregate, residential) versus "family" (biological, foster, adoptive) is not based on any psychological theory. Instead, institutional (residential) care is seen most often as a form of deficient or depriving childcare when compared to other forms of care. Care in a family (foster, kinship foster, adoptive, and, especially, biological) is presumed to be better than care in a residential situation. Of course. But why? Generally, the assumption is that children have fewer resources in residential care. Fewer emotional relationships with adults, less stimulation in their physical environment, fewer positive peer relationships, less education, and less vocational preparation. Residential care presumably also provides less stability. Yet there is no theoretical basis for unambiguous differences between the sites of care once they are unpacked in the terms of any particular theory (the characteristics of good care are described in detail in Chapter 6).

Theoretical issues are simpler when the institutional care is extreme deprivation and families are conceived as ideal havens for optimal development. In this stark view, any kind of care in groups is environmentally restrictive, emotionally unsupportive, and a setting for negative peer contagion. It is "last resort" care. Most of the research on residential care stems from theorizing at this vague level. However, we will see throughout this book that none of the theories can make unambiguous differentiations between residential care and family care. Insecure attachments occur in all types of care. Peers can have negative or positive effects on each other in all types of care. Negative and positive behaviors can be reinforced in all types of care. Children and youth experience emotional pain in all types of care. At multiple levels the environment influences behavior in all types of care. There are differences in degree that reveal distributions in any psychological characteristic or variable within each type of care and an overlap in distributions between types of care.

A common characteristic of the residential care research literature is a lack of specificity about the nature of the care children and youth receive, in groups or families. There may be a reference to staffing ratios or to a particular therapy (e.g., behavioral or psychodynamic in residential treatment centers). More often, the independent variable in experimental residential care research is a comparison of general categories of care. For example, children and youth in group care are compared to those in therapeutic foster care. Allusions may be made to the development of attachments that are made in families but not in group care. However, the specific attachment experiences of the children and youth in the two kinds of care typically are not studied. Assessments of the quality of the care are rare. This problem of specifying the nature of care in more detail has been discussed by scholars for years. McCall (2011) calls it the "unspecified" independent variable: "…the vast bulk of this literature does not specify empirically the major independent variable of interest" (p. 225). Most research on residential care is generated by general observations such as "most residential care I have seen is not very good" or even general ideological presuppositions like "children should be raised in families."

What Kinds of Inferences Can Be Made?: Research Designs

The kinds of inferences that can be made from a study's results are limited by the nature of the research design used. Descriptive or observational studies allow simple assessments of children or their environments. Researchers may want to know the distribution of ages of the residents in care. Or the educational levels of residents may be charted. Or the number of problem behaviors among children in foster care versus residential care may be counted. Descriptive studies are often helpful at the beginning of a research project to find out what is going on before more intrusive research is undertaken, but no inferences can be made about how variables are related.

Correlational studies show how one variable relates to or predicts another but do not allow causal inferences. For example, in the report of the Senate hearing described in Chapter 2, data were provided from a Children's Bureau report that documented that children and youth in residential care had more diagnosed psychological problems than children in foster care. No inference should be drawn that it was being in residential care that caused the problems, though that is often, inappropriately, the very inference that is implied or stated outright.

The only way to make causal inferences between variables (e.g., that residential care is inherently bad for children) is to use a special kind of research study, a "true experiment" or "randomized clinical trial." Research designed in this way is seen as meeting the highest standard. In technical terms, randomized clinical trials provide "internal validity"; they provide the opportunity to draw cause-effect inferences. They do so because in a true experiment, the only difference between two groups is the independent variable of interest. If groups differ after an experience or treatment, the only difference must be due to the independent variable, showing that it caused the difference. The only way to make sure that two groups are the same in every way when a study starts is to use the element of chance. A single group must be put into different groups (e.g., an "experimental group" and a "control group"—but there can be multiple kinds of experimental and/or control groups in a study) using random assignment. Every individual in the beginning sample must have an equal chance to wind up in the assigned groups. This design is used in clinical trials of drugs, medical interventions of all kinds, laboratory research with animals and humans, studies of educational methods, and many other areas where control of assignment to experimental and control groups is possible. Even in a carefully designed study, random assignment to groups at the beginning is not the only thing needed to make causal inferences possible. After assignment, it continues to be important to make sure that the groups are treated in the same way. This is difficult to do in real-world settings. Independent variables or treatments are not highly controlled events like a drug versus a placebo. As discussed in the theory section above, "residential care" versus "family care" involves complex sets of influences on children. Those two treatments differ on many dimensions and a true understanding of their relative influences on child outcomes requires an unpacking of those influences.

The "ideal" study of the effects of residential care would involve taking a large group of children or youth and randomly assigning them to stay with their families or go into residential care. Obviously, it would not be ethical to do that. There are many randomized clinical trials that pit one kind of intervention (e.g., residential care) versus another (e.g., therapeutic foster care). Some of this research is reviewed in Chapters 4 and 5. The Bucharest Early Intervention Project with Romanian infants left one randomly assigned group to stay in what were known to be extremely deprived environments to be compared to those randomly assigned to foster care provided by researcher-trained parents. That study, comparing infants sent to foster care with those who remained in an institution, will be reviewed in Chapter 4.

Because random assignment is usually impossible, some version of what is called a **quasi-experimental research design** dominates the research literature on residential care (studies using this design are common in the reviews in Chapters 4 and 5). Two or more existing groups are identified (not created by random assignment), measurements are taken over time, and trends over time in the groups are compared. However, there are serious limitations on the valid inferences that can be made from this kind of research. If a researcher compares children in foster care with those in residential care, for example, there is no way to know whether differences are due to the type of care or to systematic or unsystematic pre-existing differences in the groups. That is why this research scheme is known as "quasi-experimental" (you could call it "not really experimental"). A way to "fix" this problem is to match members of the groups on as many variables as possible. The most sophisticated form of this matching procedure in the residential care literature is called "propensity matching" and involves using computer programs to match research participants on as many variables as are available. When the number of variables used for matching is very large and the variables are very relevant to the outcomes at issue, propensity matching helps. However, the process of selection, adding and dropping participants to and from a group with matching can never guarantee equality of the groups in the way random assignment does.

Also common in residential care research is the **pretest-posttest pre-experimental design.** Children and youth are tested when they enter care and then again, perhaps upon leaving care. No comparison group, not even an unequal one, is involved. Again, no cause-effect connections can be made between residential care and outcomes. It is not a true "experiment" or even a quasi-experiment because there are so many alternative explanations for change unrelated to the residential care (the participants got older, they got better at taking the tests involved, or many of dozens of other influential events may have occurred between the pre- and posttests). It may be informative to know whether outcomes change in direction over time. Pre-post change may call into question some explanations. For example, if children and youth consistently improve on measures of positive psychological health over their time in residential care, extreme hypotheses about the inherently damaging effects of residential care are less viable.

In most of the studies reviewed in Chapters 4 and 5, there was no way to design a true experiment or randomized clinical trial. Too often, that has not prevented researchers from talking about the "effects" of residential care or some component of residential care in their studies. I am not arguing that evidence from quasi-experimental designs in residential research should be ruled out. But it must be interpreted carefully and critically. I will give just two examples to make this point. First, Ryan, Marshall, Herz, and Hernandez (2008) attempted to find a link between group home placements and the risk of delinquency. Using only archived administrative records for 8,226 adolescents, they found that adolescents who had at least one group home placement were more likely to have been arrested at some point. The study had no measures of the quality of care. It provided no data on the likelihood that those who had had a group home placement instead of a foster placement did so because they had more (or fewer) problems or had very different histories making them more or less fosterable. It did not control for differential thresholds for reports to law enforcement in family versus group home settings, among other possible differences between the groups. Yet the title of the article includes the subtitle "investigating group home *effects*" (p. 1088, my emphasis) and concludes, in causal tones, "The evidence clearly indicates that group homes significantly increase the risk of arrest" (p. 1097). Conclusions like those of Ryan et al. should not be taken at face value. Non-experimental studies that conclude "Type A care causes X" should be viewed very skeptically.

The second example of the importance of taking care in interpreting non-experimental data comes from a study in which the cause-effect implication is more subtle. It is conveyed in the emotionally laden title "I want to be there when he graduates: Foster parents show higher levels of commitment than group care providers" (Lo, Roben, Maier, Fabian, Shauffer, & Dozier, 2015). Using the My Child Interview (adapted for adolescents) to measure commitment, the investigators interviewed 31 foster parents, 18 group caregivers who worked on shifts, and 28 group caregivers who lived with youth in cottages through the week. No details on the environments are provided, but the foster care settings are described as "home-like" whereas the group care is described as "less home-like" and "more like a dorm or boarding school or even a treatment facility" (p. 96) despite an earlier description of the group care as "cottage care."

Preliminary analyses indicated that the groups differed on several variables. Foster parents were older by more than ten years than the group caregivers and caregivers rated the youth in the group settings as having more externalizing behavior problems. The commitment variable was correlated across groups with caregiver age, youth age, caregiver experience with children (negatively, i.e., higher commitment went with less experience), number of hours working with the youth, and reports of externalizing behavior (negatively, i.e., higher commitment correlated with fewer externalizing problems). The primary analysis was a comparison of group differences in commitment. Secondary analyses involved using some of the covariates (variables that were correlated with commitment) to "control" for the existing differences between the groups in age of caregiver and hours worked, but not differences in externalizing behavior or experience with children. The overall analysis of commitment showed group differences with follow-up statistics showing that foster parents had higher levels of commitment than those who worked with the youth through the week, who had higher levels than shift workers. In an analysis using youth externalizing behaviors and caregiver experience as covariates, the differences among the groups were still statistically significant, but no paired group results were reported. The authors conclude that it is not surprising that shift workers have lower commitment, but cottage care workers live with the youth and should show more commitment. "We argue that, despite attempts to make the environment somewhat home-like, the cottage care setting is nonetheless group care and not conducive to high levels of caregivers' commitment" (p. 99). The authors then buttress their argument from their data with quotations from interviews that highlight commitment differences, like the one used in the title of the article.

The problem with this study's design is that the "groups" are packages of variables that are intrinsically tied together. The statistical technique they used to "control" for group differences (analysis of covariance) cannot disentangle these ties (analysis of covariance was originally developed to adjust for random error in random assignment of participants to groups in true experiments). The foster parents were significantly older than the caregivers in the other groups (on average, in their 50s) and had much higher incomes. The authors did not mention income because the groups were not significantly different. That was likely due to the small number of participants in the study and the great variability in the shift worker incomes. However, in real purchasing power, the nearly $18,000 per year average difference between the foster parents and cottage caregivers is surely meaningful. Moreover, in their discussion section, the authors argue "Unlike shift care workers, they [cottage caregivers] did not report elevated levels of externalizing behaviors relative to foster parents" (p. 99). However, according to Table 2 (Lo et al., p. 98), cottage caregivers reported more than twice as many externalizing behaviors (4.8 to 2.2) than foster parents. The authors choose to interpret the results of their study in terms of "home-like foster care" versus "institution-like group care." But because of the quasi-experimental nature of their design and as indicated by their own data, the difference between foster caregiving and cottage caregiving easily could be interpreted as "empty-nesters with high incomes and youth with few problems" versus "cottage caregivers with their own children still at home, lower incomes, and youth to take care of who have more problems and are harder to foster." Because the nature of the study does not allow for a clear distinction between the interpretations and because the investigators undertook the study with a bias against group care, it is particularly important not to make overconfident statements about ambiguous results. The emotional content of the article's title and its discussion section are not consistent with such judiciousness.

The Global "Independent Variable": Types of Residential Care

Different kinds of residential care serve different populations of children and youth for different purposes (Arieli, Beker, & Kashti, 2000). McCall's recognition of the "unspecified independent variable" was mentioned earlier. The problem is common in reports of studies of residential care (Axford, Little, Morpeth, & Weyts, 2005; Boel-Studt & Tobia, 2016; McCall, 1999; Whittaker et al., 2016). Gunnar (2001) makes a gross distinction among "globally depriving" institutions that do not provide physical or psychological resources, institutions that provide for basic physical needs but do not provide psychological stimulation or relationships, and "psychologically depriving" institutions that provide for basic physical and environmental stimulation, but do not provide for stable, consistent relationships. Van Ijzendoorn et al. (2011) suggest a fourth level for Gunnar's system, one that provides consistent, stable caregiving. They indicate, without specific evidence, that that level of provision would be very expensive and is untypical. In residential care studies, intervention and control groups frequently combine different kinds of residential care and review articles and meta-analyses almost always examine very different forms of care without distinctions.

One way of thinking about different forms of residential care is to think about how the children and youth entered (Bellonci, Holmes, & Whittaker, 2019). Some enter through medical treatment or the mental health system, some through the juvenile justice system, and some through child welfare. Many children and youth in residential care have multiple experiences with different forms of residential care. In the research literature, distinctions are difficult to make or just not made. In the following chapters, I will be reviewing many articles with these mixtures of types of care but will start here with six different forms. Some forms are common across the world; others are found only in poorer or wealthier nations.

Institutions: The default description of care. A century and a half ago in the United States, Canada, the United Kingdom, and many other countries, children needed out-of-home care because they had lost their parents, or their single parent gave them up because they could not provide adequate care. Most of those children were placed in orphanages. Like many other kinds of 19th century institutions for those with mental illness or mental disability, orphanages were often constructed in rural areas where land was cheap and there were few neighbors to complain about their presence (Trent, 2016). Residents lived in dormitories, ate in communal halls, and worked on the institution's farms and in their laundries. Some institutions were operated by the state, others by private charities (e.g., the Masons in the United States, Webster, Wente, Parris, & Rus, 2017; Barnardo's Homes in the United Kingdom, Higginbotham, 2017).

Participants in the 1909 White House Conference on Children and Youth (Jones, 1993; *Proceedings of the Conference on the Care of Dependent Children*, 1909) called for the end of large, dreary orphanages or asylums in favor of family foster care, or, if foster care was not available, institutions organized around the "cottage plan," ideally with no more than 15–25 residents in each cottage. Similar views were proliferating throughout much of western continental Europe and other anglophone countries. Orphanages were not closed immediately because of the stress of wars and a depression on social and economic systems, but by the middle of the 20th century, large orphanages were mostly gone in North America and much of Western Europe. Why? The history is complicated, but some of the reasons are identifiable (from Jones, 1993; Smith, 1995; Smith, 2009; Webster et al., 2017): (a) From before the 1909 White House Conference, the ideology of preference for foster care over residential care was reflected in the attitudes of childcare professionals in the United States and elsewhere. Institutional care was considered inherently deficient care; (b) Governments began to provide funds to poor families (in the United States, through Aid to Families with Dependent Children provision of the 1935 Social Security Act). Poverty was the major reason families placed their children (or, often, some of their children) in care; (c) Declines in birthrates, especially after the post-second war baby boom, resulted in smaller families with more room for foster children and adoptees; (d) Because residential treatment was seen as deficient care, governments and professional organizations developed higher standards for licensure and accreditation. Requirements for professionalized staff and improved facilities raised costs dramatically, for many private providers, prohibitively. At the same time, the children and youth entering care presented with more complicated emotional and behavioral problems, also raising costs of care; and (e) In the 1950s and 1960s, a major movement toward deinstitutionalization occurred in the United States and other countries, including the United Kingdom (Fulcher, 2009). The movement was a response to scandals that got major media attention in mental hospitals (see Geller's history, Geller, 2000), facilities for those with mental disabilities (e.g., Goode, Hill, Reiss, & Bronston, 2013; Trent, 2016; Weiser, 2020), and "orphanages" (e.g., Boys Town; Kneeland, 1974). The deinstitutionalization movement was also influenced by philosophical works like those of Goffman (1961) who coined the term "total institution" in his analysis of asylums (a notion that has been widely misused in the demonization of all kinds of institutions—see Smith, 2009) and Szasz (1961) who denied that terms like "psychotic" were meaningful.

These factors, plus the enactment of legislation making adoption and fostering easier (in the United States, Adoption Assistance and Child Welfare Act of 1980 and its 1997 clarification in the Adoption and Safe Families Act, see Jones, 1993; Wilhelm, 2002) and the ratification by the United Nations of the Convention on the Rights of the Child, solidifying the centrality of the family unit and encouraging the elimination of large residential facilities led to declines in group care. But these changes did not end all group care. In North America, residential treatment care, children's homes, and group homes have continued to serve children and families (see sections on each, below). However, many studies of residential care, especially those on residential care in eastern Europe, Asia, and Africa, are conducted in "institutions." Much of the confusion about residential care can be traced to the imprecise use of the term "institution." Rather than specifying the nature of the care and parsing the differences among large institutions and other forms of care, researchers too easily describe the research site as an "institution." For example, in the recent United Kingdom Children's Commissioner (2020) report, *The children who no-one knows what to do with*, children's homes were equated with institutions on the first page of the document: "Ideally, no child should grow up in an institution." The Children's Commissioner reported there were English children who said they received love and support and were in the best place they could be, but the term "institution" has become code for "bad childcare." In a chapter in an important research monograph, van IJzendoorn et al. (2011) offer a section titled "The Nature of Institutional Care." They acknowledge the variability among institutions (for a better description of that variability, see Julian, Li, Wright, & Jimenez-Etcheverria, 2019), but refer to an "in press" publication apparently never published, presenting "...a composite description of what is typical" (p. 9) (from what follows in the chapter, an institution in Greece is the prototype, but some of the co-authors also worked with the Bucharest Early Intervention Project; the description of institutions in McCall & Groark, 2015, seems to rely on the same line of thought, but it includes more complicating conditions). The characteristics of their "typical institution" include: (a) child-adult ratios from 31:1 to 8:1 (with a few exceptions with lower ratios); (b) frequent "graduations" from one homogeneous age group to another, as many as three times in the first two or three years of life; (c) constant turnover or shuffling of staff with a child seeing up to 50–100 different caregivers in the first 19 months of life; (d) many other adults rotating through the child's space, including medical personnel and prospective adoptive parents; (e) caregivers receiving little training, especially about how to interact with children; and (f) caregivers interacting with children with little warmth or responsiveness and not encouraging exploration.

Two facts are clear from this description of the "typical institution," one that is characterized by what van IJzendoorn et al. call "structural neglect," minimal resources, unfavorable staffing, and sterile caregiver-child interactions. The first fact is that van IJzendoorn et al. are not describing any entity in the United States, the United Kingdom, Canada, or most wealthy countries in the late 20th or 21st centuries that was lawfully meeting the standards of governmental or accrediting bodies. The second fact is that they are describing institutions for very young children and infants. Confusion arises because earlier in their chapter, the authors state: "Children exposed to institutional care do not receive the type of nurturing and stimulating environment needed for normal growth and healthy psychological development" (p. 8). "Children," not "infants," "toddlers," "knee children," "preschoolers," or even "young children" (the actual subjects of their investigations). I am not nitpicking here. The authors really are talking about "institutions for infants and young children." As we will see in Chapter 4, the research findings on institutions like those described by van IJzendoorn et al. are repeatedly generalized across types of residential care, across age groups, across countries, and across time. When readers encounter research on "institutions," they should critically evaluate just what kind of environment is involved and what kinds of children or youth are experiencing it. If the term is being used in the "typical" way, it is describing very large housing units with minimal resources and little stability, and most likely, environments devoid of physical and emotional resources. It is inappropriate to generalize research results from this type of environment to other forms of residential care. Even in the same monograph in which the van IJzendoorn et al. paper appears, McCall (2011) qualifies his conclusion that "institutions are the least preferred alternative [of any rearing environment]" by saying "This may not be true of institutions for older children" (p. 255), referencing the Duke Positive Outcomes for Orphans research covered in Chapter 5. The promiscuous use of the term "institution" in the residential care research literature has been highly misleading at best and utterly destructive at worst.

Boarding schools: Educational residential care. One of the oldest forms of residential care is the boarding school (Fraser, 1968). Typically inhabited by the children of the wealthy and very wealthy, boarding schools are particularly common in the United Kingdom, the former colonies of the United Kingdom, and in the United States. Most boarding schools serve children between the ages of 12–18. Most are designed to provide high-quality academic training, but also to educate the "whole child" with emphasis on competitive sports and arts education. In the United Kingdom, boarding schools are used by parents in the upper classes to create elite educational environments and socialization and networking (old school ties) opportunities for future employment in the private and governmental sectors, traditionally for males, but increasingly for females too. In the United States, boarding schools are used by parents to prepare their children for elite post-secondary education. At Ivy league universities and schools like Georgetown, Duke, and Stanford, students who attended boarding schools are admitted at a rate considerably above their representation in the population (Persell, Catsambis, & Cookson, 1992). American parents also use boarding schools as elite educational alternatives to the public and private day schools they consider insufficiently strong to prepare their children for success. Boarding schools, particularly military schools, have also been used by wealthy families to deal with offspring with behavior problems. Biographies of the rich and famous, including presidents, prime ministers, and CEOs, frequently refer to their boarding school experiences (good and bad) as instrumental in their development.

Interestingly, there is little beyond anecdotal evidence about the effectiveness of boarding schools. Cookson (2009) concludes that the boarding schools are "...virtually invisible to policymakers and the general public..." and "seldom researched" (p. 462). Of the most elite boarding schools in the United States, he further concludes that they "...have closed their gates to the prying eyes of outside researchers" (Cookson, 2009; p. 463). In both the United Kingdom and the United States, elite boarding schools often are deemed to provide the best education money can buy. Consumer satisfaction ratings are in the 90th percentiles. However, there is ambivalence about boarding schools. In the United Kingdom, many of the nation's leaders are graduates of elite boarding schools. Yet, critics argue that the boarding school experience develops leaders with flawed personalities. Schaverien (2004, 2011), based on her own clinical experience with adults who are former boarding school residents, identifies what she calls "boarding school syndrome." A Jungian analyst, Schaverien's evidence for the syndrome comes largely from case studies. Working backward from adults who have difficulty forming social relationships, she argues that individuals separated from their families and without close adult relationships have a form of attachment disorder that is exacerbated by frequent bullying by peers. The resulting syndrome includes a loose set of symptoms including homesickness, a sense of loss of freedom, and homelessness during the boarding experience and a subsequent continuing lack of intimacy in adulthood. In Britain, children in foster care are called "looked after children or youth" or "children in care." Schaverien concludes that those labels fit residents in boarding schools.

Nevertheless, unlike other forms of residential care, for families, boarding schools are preferred options, not last resorts. While group care for the poor, the abandoned, and the abused has fallen into disrepute, elite boarding schools have continued to thrive, despite astronomical costs. In an overview chapter on residential care, Lee (2020) suggests that youth of lesser means should have access to educational residential care. She argues that there need to be more institutions like the Milton Hershey School in Pennsylvania (serving 2,000 children and youth from pre-kindergarten through high school) and the Pasqual Academy in California. Lee argues that "what works for whom in residential education remains unknown" yet she also says "...the potential for boarding schools to provide a high-quality educational experience for privileged youth is well established" (Lee, p. 315). Indeed, if the yardstick for effectiveness is the likelihood of attending a highly ranked college or university, rather than some broader version of developmental health, it is hard to argue against boarding schools (although if the histories of boarding schools designed to force the acculturation of native populations in the United States and Canada is considered, the conclusion is quite different, Gray & Cote, 2019; Stout, 2012; Woolford, 2015). The contrast between the assumed effectiveness of the boarding school and the assumed dangers of the "orphanage" environment could not be more striking. Perhaps the difference is based on the ability of the privileged residents to visit their families on holidays and in summers, although the large number of summer camps in which highly privileged youth spend their whole summers suggests that that contact may be limited. For the denizens of boarding schools, life after the early elementary school years may be one where very little time is spent at "home."

The Boarding School's upper-class students are too different from those who reside in residential care like children's homes to learn much from them for the purposes of this book. However, in some ways the boarding school environment is more like the modern children's home environment than other forms of residential care or the stereotypical institution. Perhaps it is ironic that one of the innovations in foster care in recent years has been the development of residential programs (often called "independent living programs" or "academies") for those aging out of care (e.g., Doucet, Greeson, & Eldeeb, 2022).

Custodial care: Residential care for youth offenders. The most restrictive version of residential care is provided for young law breakers. They are variously called (sometimes euphemistically) reform schools, training schools, youth detention centers, or even junior jails. Their histories are often state-specific. Across states and countries, their nature and use are subject to how the "law and order" political winds are blowing (Billitteri, 2010; Reuterman & Hughes, 1984). At some point in their histories, most governments used some rather draconian form of large institution for housing juvenile offenders. However, the general deinstitutionalization trends of the 1970s led many states to explore alternatives to large prison-like institutions and extremely restrictive housing for all but the most dangerous youth, including "boot camps," wilderness programs, group homes, in-home interventions, or supervised probation. Most young people in youth detention are there because of non-violent offenses (Mendel, 2011).

The purported aim of this form of residential care is to rehabilitate the offender, or, at least, to reduce recidivism and to protect the community from dangerous actors. The single outcome measure used in most research with juvenile offenders is some indicator of recidivism. Avoiding custody is success; returning to custody is failure. Meta-analyses (statistical aggregations across many studies) of the effects of custodial care have revealed that restrictive versions of custodial care do not reduce recidivism (Billitteri, 2010; Lipsey, 2009; Loughran et al., 2009). Moreover, there is evidence that youth learn worse behaviors by being housed with other offenders without appropriate supervision (the "iatrogenic effect", Mendel, 2011—but see Chapter 4). Interventions that do work focus on cognitive-behavioral therapy, skill development, and education (Henggeler & Schoenwald, 2011) and do not employ large prison-like settings.

Custodial forms of care, like boarding schools, have little in common with the focus of this book. However, we occasionally will consider research on custodial care when research studies include group homes that have been used as an alternative to traditional youth detention (e.g., group homes frequently have been used in research conducted in California). It is unlikely that any of the usual or reform versions of custodial care would come close to conforming to the high-quality residential care characteristics described in Chapter 6 of this book. Although I believe that The Annie E. Casey Foundation has not made a research-based case against residential care of all kinds, they arguably are on firmer ground regarding custodial care (Mendel, 2011). That is not surprising because whereas good residential care for nonoffenders is based on strong developmental principles, typical custodial care is not. Much of the research on custodial care concerns the iatrogenic effect, the commonsensical notion that if troubled children and youth who are acting out are housed without appropriate supervisory structure with other aggressive children and youth, their behavior is likely to worsen.

Residential treatment centers: Therapeutic residential care. Early in the 20th century, Lightner Witmer and other psychologists started clinics to assess children who were struggling in school (Witmer is given credit for starting "clinical" psychology). These "child guidance" clinics stressed testing designed to identify the child's strengths and weaknesses (Witmer, 1907/1996). They typically did not provide interventions to ameliorate problems. These children also did not belong in asylums or mental hospitals, training schools, orphanages, or other kinds of institutions. During the 1930s and 1940s, psychiatrists created special residential centers for the increasing number of children with vague diagnoses such as "emotional disturbance" or "delinquency." These new treatment centers, many with private funding, used a mixture of techniques from the mental hygiene movement (Beers, 1910) and psychoanalytic therapy to develop a treatment model (see Doroshow, 2019, for a detailed history of residential treatment centers). Its components included psychotherapy, casework with the child's parents, and what was called the "therapeutic milieu." The milieu, following Freudian and neo-Freudian principles, provided a residential environment that was warm, welcoming, and permissive. The individual psychotherapy provided ranged from an hour a day to as little as an hour a week in some centers.

Therapeutic residential treatment centers grew in number through the 1940s and into the 1960s. Many traditional orphanages morphed into treatment centers. The treatment models often changed from psychoanalytic to behavioral or cognitive behavioral and some centers added day-treatment and foster care components as part of a continuum of care. Starting in the late 1960s, residential centers were subject to the criticisms of the deinstitutionalization movement and the philosophical emphasis on families being the only proper place for children and youth. Critics also raised questions about the effectiveness and cost of residential care. Increasingly, care was provided for the most severely disturbed children and youth (those who had been "leveled" or "sectioned" due to diagnoses such as severe depression, schizophrenia, or serious conduct disorders). Periods in residence got shorter and work with families got more attention.

In 2016, a group of therapeutic residential care advocates from around the world (Whittaker et al., 2016) met to regain momentum for therapeutic residential care by developing a consensus statement on the nature of and need for therapeutic care in residential settings. The working group recognizes the lack of research on treatment effectiveness and the problems of cost. They also assert the need for residential care for some children and youth and the need to work in concert with families. Their principles include a vision of partnership with parents and professionals embedded in the child's community, culture, and social relationships. They stress "learning through living" (harkening back to the therapeutic milieu) and teaching "in a series of deeply personal, human relationships" (Whittaker et al., 2016, p. 97). They see as essential the identification of evidence-based models that are effective, replicable, and scalable.

Therapeutic residential care centers are difficult to distinguish from children's homes. Both forms of care are therapeutic, both as research descriptors and in practice. Two features of therapeutic residential care sites distinguish them. First, therapeutic residential care centers are designed for children and youth displaying behavioral or emotional problems so severe that they are dangers to themselves, their families, or their communities. If individuals have broken the law, their care is likely to look more like, or occur in, custodial care. Second, although family situations are always involved, the core purpose of residential treatment follows the medical model. Something is wrong with the child or youth, and they must be treated. Most children in the United States referred for therapeutic residential care have experienced multiple hospital placements and interventions while living at home prior to placement (Bellonci et al., 2019). However, residential treatment is not hospitalization (Leichtman, 2006). Many children in therapeutic residential care have siblings who do not need to be treated. Therapeutic residential care centers and children's homes and group homes of high quality will share many features as will be apparent in Chapter 6.

Group homes: Housing children and youth in the community. In the United States, as part of the historical deinstitutionalization process, the Community Mental Health Act of 1963 provided funds to "catchment areas" (usually clusters of counties) to develop community-based mental health programming as institutions, sometimes very large ones, closed by the score (Erickson, 2021). Similar processes occurred throughout the anglophone countries (Whittaker, Holmes, del Valle, & James, 2023). One way communities dealt with former residents of various types of institutions, including orphanages, was to develop "group homes" or "halfway houses." Many group homes for children and youth were affiliated with institutions that were once orphanages or had become children's homes or private agencies with their roots in older institutions. Most group homes are relatively small, housing four to eight residents. Some are staffed by well-trained, professional staff. Many, however, are staffed by very young, inexperienced staff who are not much older than the residents (they provide a common entry-level position for graduates with a bachelor's degree in psychology or sociology). Staff turnover is a common problem. Group homes have the advantage of being in the communities where residents' families are (although that can also cause problems) but often have the disadvantage of limited access to recreational, educational, and counseling services.

Deinstitutionalization created a debate in mental health that has continued for more than four decades. Some critics (e.g., Perry, 2016) have argued that residents of the old state mental hospitals (that had been called "snake pits") moved to another institution, group homes, run by private agencies at a profit ("cash cows") that did not provide meaningful services. Other critics (e.g., Dear & Wolch, 1987; Nasrallah, 2008; Paulson, 2012), without disputing the fact that bad institutions should have been closed or radically reformed, suggest that there are many unintended consequences in the closing of the state mental hospitals, including increased homelessness, prison incarcerations, and family dysfunction. There has been less debate about closing institutions for children, perhaps because many of the more institutional characteristics of the old orphanages (e.g., barracks living) were gone by 1960s, or, more likely, because they were simply lumped in the vague category of "institutions."

Children's homes: Protective/developmental residential care. Over the past 50–80 years, many small "institutions" that were once orphanages closed, morphed into different kinds of children's services, or became children's homes. Often privately supported or using mixed private and public funds, the children's homes provide a family-like place to live for children and youth for whom "family" has not worked. Young people stay in these homes for a few months, a few years, or until they are ready for family reunification, family foster care, adoption, or independent forms of living. Unlike institutions, they provide smaller adult-to-child ratios, more staff stability, more resources, and more focus on individual children and their development. Unlike treatment facilities, they are not designed to "fix" a child or youth with severe and particular emotional or behavioral problems. High-quality homes are not holding places, but a form of treatment, with the best ones adhering to a treatment model (see the examples of models in Chapter 7). Unlike custodial care, residents are not offenders (although they may have been at one time). Instead, they are often wards of the court. It is their families that have been offenders in most cases. Their families may be engaged in illegal activities such as drug or sex trafficking or have been neglectful or abusive.

Modern children's homes, especially those in the United States, typically include residential care as one component of a constellation of care that may include emergency foster care for very young children, foster care training and placement services, adoption services, family preservation services, and independent living and transitional living programs for young adults who have aged out of the foster system or are about to do so. The main function of the children's home is to provide stability and resources to children and youth who have had neither in their developmental histories. When a houseparent model is used, and even when shift workers are consistent, children and youth can develop long-term relationships with caregivers and peers (Ayotte, Lanctôt, & Tourigny, 2015). They receive educational support (either in local public schools, or, on larger campuses, in their own schools). Because many residents in children's homes have experienced multiple out-of-home placements, they have checkered education histories and need extra support. They also have opportunities for counseling and therapy as needed, regular medical care, recreational and vocational training opportunities, and when possible, therapeutic, supervised connections with families of origin. Older residents of children's homes may stay at the home until they become independent adults. Younger residents may spend a year or two or three (depending on the vagaries of the involved social agencies and the resident's needs) before entering a foster care home or being adopted when the rights of parents of origin have been revoked. Unlike the Hollywood *Little Rascals* or *Little Orphan Annie* or Dickensian depictions of children's homes, good modern homes provide the stability and resources described by Richard McKenzie (1996) in his memoir and by the hundreds of alumni he has contacted over the years (see Chapter 5).

Versions of the independent variable: Summary. When studies compare residential care to some form of family care, the nature of the residential care is rarely specified (in many cases, nor is the family care). In many studies, there is a mix of forms of care, even when treatment is supposed to be based on a particular form of therapy (Bettmann & Jasperson, 2009). For example, children and youth from some form of group home and therapeutic residential care or group home and children's homes are often studied in the same project. More problematic is the ease with which some scholars and policy makers have generalized results from research in one kind of setting to other settings. Most problematic of all has been the frequent generalization of results from studies of large, understaffed, under-resourced institutions to therapeutic residential centers or children's homes. Combined with problems of sampling the children studied (see below), generalizations about residential care research have often been highly misleading.

What Is Being Measured?: Child Outcomes

Perhaps the most important component of a research study is what is being observed or measured. The investigator wants to know *about* something. How are the children or youth in residential care doing, physically, psychologically, behaviorally, educationally, vocationally? The central meaning of research on residential care will be found in what is measured or observed. Psychologists and other social scientists call what they are measuring "constructs." The term suggests that what are being studied are not objects of nature lying around the environment, but theoretical constructions of the investigators. For the research to be meaningful the constructs being used must have "construct validity." Construct validity cannot be summed up in a number or single judgment. Establishing construct validity is a process (Cronbach & Meehl, 1955). It involves the statement of clear definitions of the construct, the development of multiple measurement instruments, assessing how the construct relates to other constructs it should be related to (convergent validity) and is not related to other constructs it should not be related to (discriminant validity), how the construct changes over time or age, and many other factors.

For example, a frequently used construct in residential care literature, especially some of the earliest studies and of the youngest children (Zeanah, Smyke, & Settles, 2006), is intelligence. Establishing the construct validity of intelligence has been a century and a half process that is still not completed to the satisfaction of many (e.g., Murdoch, 2007; Robson, 2019; Staub, 2018). In the residential care literature, intelligence has been used as a general indicator of cognitive development since the mid-20th century studies. If residences, as deprived environments, have negative influences on development, the assumption is that those negative influences will show up in the form of lower intelligence scores. A wide variety of intelligence tests have been used in the research on residential care. Among them are well-established tests like the various Weschler scales and the Stanford-Binet. So-called infant intelligence scales have been used with infants and young children in care (e.g., the Bayley Scales, the Merrill-Palmer, versions of the McCarthy scales). Intelligence tests for older children and youth have been shown to be predictive of school achievement. Infant intelligence scores have not been shown to be highly predictive of much of anything after the age of two. When you are reading the residential care literature, it is important to keep in mind what measures are being used and the limits on what they can tell you. Here are the major types of measures commonly used in residential care research (references are examples of studies using the type of measurement).

Direct observations or reports. Included in this category are simple measures of physical development, including height, weight, body mass, indicators of educational success, such as highest grade attained or high school graduation, and placement status, such as returning to family of origin, entry into foster care, or number of placements. Other indicators may come from archival files, like alcohol use, drug use, smoking, or contact with biological parents (e.g., Duppong Hurley, Lambert, Gross, Thompson, & Farmer, 2017; Gross et al., 2015). In studies of youth in the juvenile justice system, measures might include number of misdemeanor or felony charges, or other indicators of involvement with law enforcement. Information about the child's environment may also be observed directly, including staff/child ratios, availability of toys and books, recreational opportunities staff turnover, etc. The most respected measurement in child development research involves the use of behavioral observations. For example, if you are studying bullying, you define subcategories of bullying in behavioral terms, minimizing subjectivity (and thus increasing inter-observer agreement), and then do counts of how often the behaviors occur. Behavioral observations are rare in the residential care literature, probably due to expense and ethical (intrusiveness) concerns.

Behavioral ratings and checklists. Ratings of behavior by caregivers, parents, teachers, peers, and others are much more common in residential care research than direct behavioral observations. Frequently used measures include standardized versions of rating scales, including the Assessment Checklist for Children, Child Behavior Checklist, the Children's Global Assessment Scale, and the Behavior Assessment Scale for Children. Some ratings have forms for teachers, parents/caregivers, and peers to complete. Investigators may develop their own rating forms or modify available ones for specific studies. Ratings introduce a degree of subjectivity that can raise questions about their reliability and validity. However, they are much cheaper and easier to use than direct observations (e.g., Tarren-Sweeney, 2007). Investigators generally are aware of the problems with ratings and often point out that when they use multiple raters (e.g., teachers and parents or caregivers), the raters often do not agree about the same child.

Interviews. Interviews with children and youth, parents, and caregivers are common in the residential care literature. They can provide detailed pictures about what is going on. However, conducting interviews is expensive in time and money. Reducing the results of interviews to communicable units of information is difficult. An hour-long interview can require many hours of labor-intensive analysis (e.g., Anglin, 2011; Fischer, Dölitzsch, Schmeck, Fegert, & Schmid, 2016; Neagu & Sebba, 2019). Interviews usually occur in small-scale studies, raising questions about applying the findings to other populations and settings.

Self-reports and surveys. Along with ratings, self-reports are among the most common measures used in residential care research. The child versions of some of the checklists listed above are self-reports of the same behaviors being rated by parents and teachers. Residents often are asked about their self-perceptions in measures like the International Survey of Children's Well-Being the Personal Well-Being Index—School Children, the Overall Life Satisfaction (OLS) scale, and the Questionnaire for Youth in Residential Care. Other surveys may ask about group climate, maltreatment, or motivation (e.g., Attar-Schwartz, 2019; Holden & Sellers, 2019; Nijhof, Veerman, Engels, & Scholte, 2011; Steinke & Derrick, 2018).

Standardized tests. The most commonly used standardized tests in the residential care literature are intelligence tests, as discussed above. Educational achievement tests also are common, usually administered by schools, not investigators. For infants and young children, there are standardized means for assessing attachment security, including the Attachment Q-sort and the Attachment Story Completion Task (e.g., Sparling, Dragomir, Ramey, & Florescu, 2005; Zeanah et al., 2006).

Neurological and physiological measures. Recently there has been increased interest in using measures of brain functioning and stress (cortisol measures, telomere length, and even a standardized procedure, the Trier Social Stress Test). These have not been used extensively in the residential care research literature but have been included in the Bucharest Early Intervention Project's work, described in Chapter 4 (e.g., Humphreys et al., 2016).

Regardless of the kinds of measure used, it is important that they be accurate and stable (i.e., reliable) and meaningful (i.e., valid). With the growing focus on "evidence-based" practices, it is essential that the evidence is good. The absence of direct behavioral observations in much of the research is unfortunate but understandable. Using measures with the lowest possible degree of inference and bias is advantageous. Most dependent variables are open to criticism of some kind. However, in residential care research, the problems with dependent variables do not appear to be as great as those with independent variables or generalization.

To Whom Do the Results Apply?: The Generalization Problem

In addition to the theoretical questions, research designs, and measures, the other major component of a research study is the sample or samples being studied. There is much variability in the samples used on research in the United States and the variability increases exponentially when the international literature is considered (James, 2023; Whittaker et al., 2016). The ideal sampling approach is to carefully identify a population and then randomly choose a reasonably large number of individuals from the identified population (there are formulas for making decisions about sample size). The point of randomness here is to insure representativeness. The technical term for making solid inferences about generalization is "external validity." There need to be methodological and theoretical bases for generalization (Findley, Kikuta, & Denly, 2021; Lucas, 2003). It is important to distinguish random sampling and random assignment. The former deals with the groups the inferences from a study can be generalized to (external validity). The latter deals with the study design and what kinds of inferences are appropriate (causal or correlational—internal validity).

Although random sampling is the ideal sampling method, it is rarely used in the research reviewed in this book. It is difficult to precisely define the population of children to be sampled from. Even if that was done, for example, "children and youth referred for care in California in a three-year period," choosing a truly representative group for such a population would be prohibitively expensive (and seldom is research in this area lavishly funded). Most studies use "convenience sampling." You study those who are available to you. In the strictest sense, your findings are not generalizable to any other group because no other group would have the same characteristics as the group that was available to you. There may be peculiarities to your sample that make them unique. Due to this limitation, results should be cautiously generalized. One way that researchers can gain more confidence in research from convenience samples is to replicate research in different groups and settings. When the same findings are obtained in research in a variety of populations and settings, it becomes more reasonable to infer that a treatment or intervention applies within and across populations. A good example is research on the Teaching Family Model that is examined in Chapter 7. The Teaching Family Model has been used successfully with so many populations in so many settings that its effectiveness is well established despite the use of samples of convenience in most studies of it.

The question of whom results can be applied to is central to the main argument in this book. Residential care is frequently condemned based on research on age groups and populations and in settings that are not representative. The most egregious instances of overgeneralization are found in the application of the research findings on infants and young children reared in extremely deprived environments in Romania to older children and youth in very different settings in developed countries where such care for infants and young children in extreme environments has been rare for more than half a century.

Summary: What to Look for in Reading Research on Residential Care

Here are some questions to keep in mind when considering the research literature on residential care. What questions, theoretical or practical, are being addressed? What meaningful constructs are being studied and are their measures reliable and valid? How is the research designed? What limitations are put on the nature of the inferences that can be made using that design? What do we know about the residential care and comparison settings being studied? Finally, and perhaps most important, to what groups of children in what settings is it legitimate to generalize? This is the critical framework that will be used in evaluating the research considered in Chapters 4 through 7.

References

Anglin, J. P. (2011). *Translating the Cornell CARE program model into practice: Lessons from the pioneer agencies on changing agency cultures and care practice.* Retrieved from: http://rccp.cornell.edu/_assets/Translating%20the%20CARE%20Program%20Model%20into%20Practice%20James%20Anglin.pdf.

Arieli, M., Beker, J., & Kashti, Y. (2000). Residential group care as a socializing environment: Toward a broader perspective. *Child and Youth Care Forum, 30*, 403–414. doi: 10.1023/A:1015321302983.

Attar-Schwartz, S. (2019). Parental availability of support and frequency of contact: The reports of youth in educational residential care. *Children and Youth Services Review, 101*, 317–328. doi: 10.1016/j.childyouth.2019.04.016.

Axford, N., Little, M., Morpeth, L., & Weyts, A. (2005). Evaluating children's services: Recent conceptual and methodological developments. *British Journal of Social Work, 35*, 73–88. doi: 10.1093/bjsw/bch163.

Ayotte, M.-H., Lanctôt, N., & Tourigny, M. (2015). Pre-treatment profiles of adolescent girls as predictors of the strength of their working alliances with practitioners in residential care settings. *Children and Youth Services Review, 53*, 61–69. doi: 10.1016/j.childyouth.2015.03.010.

Bauer, H. H. (1992). *Scientific literacy and the myth of the scientific method.* Urbana: University of Illinois Press.

Beers, C. W. (1910). *A mind that focused itself: An autobiography* (2nd ed.). New York: Longmans, Green.

Bellonci, C., Holmes, L., & Whittaker, J. K. (2019). Re-thinking therapeutic residential care (TRC) as a preventive service: Examining developments in the US and England. *Residential Treatment for Children & Youth*, *36*, 35–53. doi: 10.1080/0886571X.2018.1536495.

Bettmann, J. E., & Jasperson, R. A. (2009). Adolescents in residential and inpatient treatment: A review of the outcome literature. *Child & Youth Care Forum*, *38*, 161–183. doi: 10.1007/s10566-009-9073-y.

Billitteri, T. J. (2010). Youth violence: The issues. *CQ Researcher*, *20* (March), 195–201. Retrieved from: https://cqpress.sagepub.com/cqresearcher/report/youth-violence-cqresrre20100305.

Boel-Studt, S. M., & Tobia, L. (2016). A review of trends, research, and recommendations for strengthening the evidence-base and quality of residential group care. *Residential Treatment for Children & Youth*, *33*, 13–35. doi:10.1080/0886571X.2016.1175995.

Children's Commissioner. (2020). *The children who no-one knows what to do with*. Retrieved from: https://www.childrenscommissioner.gov.uk/wp-content/uploads/2020/11/cco-the-children-who-no-one-knows-what-to-do-with/.

Cookson, P. W. (2009). Perspectives on elite boarding schools. In M. Berends, M. G. Springer, D. Ballou, & H. J. Walberg (Eds.), *Handbook of research on school choice* (pp. 461–478). New York: Routledge.

Cronbach, L. J., & Meehl, P. E. (1955). Construct validity in psychological tests. *Psychological Bulletin*, *52*, 281–302. doi: 10.1037/h0040957.

Dear, M. J., & Wolch, J. R. (1987). *Landscapes of despair: From deinstitutionalization to homelessness*. Princeton, NJ: Princeton University Press.

Doroshow, D. B. (2019). *Emotionally disturbed: A history of caring for America's troubled children*. Chicago, IL: University of Chicago Press.

Doucet, M. M., Greeson, J. K. P., & Eldeeb, N. (2022). Independent living programs and services for youth 'aging out' of care in Canada and the U. S.: A systematic review. *Children and Youth Services Review*, *142*, 106630. doi: 10.1016/j.childyouth.2022.106630.

Duppong Hurley, K. D., Lambert, M. C., Gross, T. J., Thompson, R. W., & Farmer, E. M. Z. (2017). The role of therapeutic alliance and fidelity in predicting youth outcomes during therapeutic residential care. *Journal of Emotional and Behavioral Disorders*, *25*, 37–45. doi: 10.1177/1063426616686756.

Erickson, B. (2021, June). Deinstitutionalization through optimism: The Community Mental Health Act of 1963. *The American Journal of Psychiatry Residents' Journal*, 6–7. doi: 10.1176/appi.ajp-rj.2021.160404.

Findley, M. G., Kikuta, K., & Denly, M. (2021). External validity. *Annual Review of Political Science*, *24*, 365–393. doi: 10.1146/annurev-polisci-041719-102556.

Fischer, S., Dölitzsch, C., Schmeck, K., Fegert, J. M., & Schmid, M. (2016). Interpersonal trauma and associated psychopathology in girls and boys living in residential care. *Children and Youth Services Review*, *67*, 203–211. doi: 10.1016/j.childyouth.2016.06.013.

Fraser, W. R. (1968). *Residential education*. Oxford: Pergamon Press.

Fulcher, L. C. (2009). Foreword. In M. Smith (Ed.), *Rethinking residential child care: Positive perspectives*. Bristol: Policy Press.

Geller, J. L. (2000). The last half-century of psychiatric services as reflected in *Psychiatric Services*. *Psychiatric Service*, *51*, 41–67. doi: 10.1176/ps.51.1.41.

Goffman, E. (1961). *Asylums: Essays on the social situation of mental patients and other inmates*. Chicago, IL: Aldine Publishing.

Goode, D., Hill, D. B., Reiss, J., & Bronston, W. (2013). *A history and sociology of the Willowbrook State School*. Washington, DC: American Association on Intellectual and Developmental Disabilities.

Gray, A. P., & Cote, W. (2019). Cultural connectedness protects mental health against the effect of historical trauma among Anishinabe young adults. *Public Health*, *176*, 77–81. doi: 10.1016/j.puhe.2018.12.003.

Gross, T. J., Duppong Hurley, K. D., Sullivan, J. J., Lambert, M. C., van Ryzin, M. J., & Thompson, R. W. (2015). Program records as a source for program implementation assessment and youth outcomes predictors during residential care. *Children and Youth Services Review*, *58*, 153–162. doi: 10.1016/j.childyouth.2015.09.016.

Gunnar, M. (2001). Effects of early deprivation. In C. A. Nelson & M. Luciana (Eds.), *Handbook of developmental neuroscience* (pp. 617–629). Cambridge: MIT Press.

Henggeler, S., & Schoenwald, S. J. (2011). Evidence-based interventions for juvenile offenders and juvenile justice policies that support them. *SRCD Social Policy Report*, *25*(1), 1–20. doi: 10.1002/j.2379-3988.2011.tb00066.x.

Higginbotham, P. (2017). *Children's homes: A history of institutional care for Britain's young*. Barnsley: Pen & Sword History.

Holden, M. J., & Sellers, D. E. (2019). An evidence-based program model for facilitating therapeutic responses to pain-based behavior in residential care. *International Journal of Child, Youth and Family Studies*, *10*, 63–80. doi: 10.18357/ijcyfs102-3201918853.

Humphreys, K. L., Esteves, K., Zeanah, K., Fox, N. A., Nelson III, C. A., & Drury, S. S. (2016). Accelerated telomere shortening: Tracking the lasting impact of early institutional care at the cellular level. *Psychiatry Research*, *246*, 95–100. doi: 10.1016/j.psychres.2016.09.023.

James, S. (2023). A cross-national comparison of residential care for children and youth: Conceptual and methodological foundations. In J. K. Whittaker, L. Holmes, J. F. del Valle, & S. James (Eds.), *Revitalizing residential care for children and youth: Cross-national trends and challenges* (pp. 25–40). New York: Oxford University Press. doi: 10.1093/oso/9780197644300.003.0003.

Jones, M. B. (1993). Decline of the American orphanage, 1941-1980. *Social Services Review*, *67*, 459–480. doi: 10.1086/603999.

Julian, M. M., Li, J., Wright, A., & Jimenez-Etcheverria, P. A. (2019). Young children in institutional care: Characteristics of institutions, children's development, and interventions. In T. Tulviste, D. L. Best, & J. L. Gibbons (Eds.), *Children's social worlds in cultural context* (pp. 217–229). Cham: Springer. doi: 10.1007/978-3-030-27033-9_16.

Kneeland, D. E. (1974, April 16). Boys Town has an embarrassment of riches. *New York Times*, p. 41.

Laudan, L. (1977). *Progress and its problems: Toward a theory of scientific growth*. Berkeley: University of California Press.

Lee, B. R. (2020). Residential programs: Opportunities and challenges in the 21st-century treatment environment. In T. W. Farmer, M. A. Conroy, E. M. Z. Farmer, & K. S. Sutherland (Eds.), *Handbook of research on emotional and behavioral disorders: Interdisciplinary developmental perspectives on children and youth* (pp. 306–320). New York: Routledge. doi: 10.4324/9780429453106-21.

Leichtman, M. (2006). Residential treatment of children and adolescents: Past, present, and future. *American Journal of Orthopsychiatry*, *76*, 285–294. doi: 10.1037/0002-9432.76.3.285.

Lipsey, M. W. (2009). The primary factors that characterize effective interventions with juvenile offenders: A meta-analytic overview. *Victims & Offenders*, *4*, 124–147. doi: 10.1080/15564880802612573.

Lo, A., Roben, C. K. P., Maier, C., Fabian, K., Shauffer, C., & Dozier, M. (2015). "I want to be there when he graduates:" Foster parents show higher levels of commitment than group care providers. *Children and Youth Services Review*, *51*, 95–100. doi: 10.1016/j.childyouth.2015.01.022.

Loughran, T. A., Mulvey, E. P., Schubert, C. A., Fagan, J., Piquero, A. R., & Losoya, S. H. (2009). Estimating a dose-response relationship between length of stay and future recidivism in serious juvenile offenders. *Criminology*, *47*, 699–740. doi: 10.1111/j.1745-9125.2009.00165.x.

Lucas, J. W. (2003). Theory-testing, generalization, and the problem of external validity. *Sociological Theory*, *21*, 236–253. doi: 10.1111/1467-9558.00187.

McCall, J. N. (1999). Research on the psychological effects of orphanage care: A critical review. In R. B. McKenzie (Ed.), *Rethinking orphanages in the 21st century* (pp. 127–150). Thousand Oaks, CA: Sage.

McCall, R. B. (2011). Research, practice, and policy perspectives on issues of children without permanent parental care. In R. B. McCall, M. H. van IJzendoorn, F. Juffer, C. J. Groark, & V. K. Groza (Eds.), Children without permanent parents: Research, practice, and policy. *Monographs of the Society for Research in Child Development*, *76*(4), 223–272. doi: 10.1111/j.1540-5834.2011.00626.x.

McCall, R. B., & Groark, C. J. (2015). Research on institutionalized children: Implications for international child welfare practitioners and policymakers. *International Perspectives in Psychology: Research, Practice, Consultation*, 4, 142–159. doi: 10.1037/ipp0000033.

McKenzie, R. B. (1996). *The Home: A memoir of growing up in an orphanage*. New York: Basic.

Mendel, R. A. (2011). *No place for kids: The case for reducing juvenile incarceration*. Baltimore, MD: Annie E. Casey Foundation. Retrieved from: https://assets.aecf.org/m/resourcedoc/aecf-NoPlaceForKidsFullReport-2011.pdf.

Murdoch, S. (2007). *IQ: A smart history of a failed idea*. Hoboken, NJ: Wiley.

Nasrallah, H. A. (2008). Bring back the asylums? The tragic consequences of deinstitutionalization. *Current Psychiatry*, 7, 19–20. Retrieved from: https://link.gale.com/apps/doc/A177183702/HRCA?u=anon~a8e6a5bb&sid=googleScholar&xid=6f54e746.

Neagu, M., & Sebba, J. (2019). Who do they think they are: Making sense of self in residential care, foster care, and adoption. *Children and Youth Services Review*, *105*, 104449. doi: 10.1016/j.childyouth.2019.104449.

Nijhof, K. S., Veerman, J. W., Engels, R. C. M. E., & Scholte, R. H. J. (2011). Compulsory residential care: An examination of treatment improvement of individual and family functioning. *Children and Youth Services Review*, *33*, 1779–1785. doi: 10.1016/j.childyouth.2011.05.001.

Paulson, G. W. (2012). *Closing the asylums: Causes and consequences of the deinstitutionalization movement*. Jefferson, NC: McFarland.

Perry, B. L. (Ed.). (2016). *50 years after deinstitutionalization: Mental illness in contemporary communities*. Bingley: Emerald.

Persell, C. H., Catsambis, S., & Cookson, P. W. Jr. (1992). Family background, school type, and college attendance: A conjoint system of cultural capital transmission. *Journal of Research on Adolescence*, 2, 1–23. doi: 10.1207/s15327795jra0201_1.

Proceedings of the Conference on the Care of Dependent Children. (1909). Washington, DC: Government Printing Office.

Reuterman, N. A., & Hughes, T. R. (1984). Developments in juvenile justice during the decade of the 70s: Juvenile detention facilities. *Journal of Criminal Justice*, *12*, 325–333. doi: 10.1016/0047-2352(84)90046-1.

Robson, D. (2019). *The intelligence trap: Why smart people make dumb mistakes*. New York: Norton.

Ryan, J. P., Marshall, J. M., Herz, D., & Hernandez, P. M. (2008). Juvenile delinquency in child welfare: Investigating group home effects. *Children and Youth Services Review*, *30*, 1088–1099. doi: 10.1016/j.childyouth.2008.02.004.

Schaverien, J. (2004). Boarding school: The trauma of the "privileged" child. *Journal of Analytical Psychology*, *49*, 683–705. doi: 10.1111/j.0021-8774.2004.00495.x.

Schaverien, J. (2011). Boarding school syndrome: Broken attachments a hidden trauma. *British Journal of Psychotherapy*, *27*, 138–155. doi: 10.1111/j.1752-0118.2011.01229.x.

Smith, E. P. (1995). Bring back the orphanages?: What policymakers of today can learn from the past. *Child Welfare*, *74*, 115–142. Retrieved from: https://link.gale.com/apps/doc/A177183702/HRCA?u=anon~a8e6a5bb&sid=googleScholar&xid=6f54e746.

Smith, M. (2009). *Rethinking residential care: Positive perspectives*. Bristol: The Policy Press.

Sparling, J., Dragomir, C., Ramey, S. L., & Florescu, L. (2005). An educational intervention improves developmental progress of young children in a Romanian orphanage. *Infant Mental Health Journal*, 26, 127–142. doi: 10.1002/imhj.20040.

Staub, M. E. (2018). *The mismeasure of minds: Debating race and intelligence between Brown and The Bell Curve*. Chapel Hill: University of North Carolina Press.

Steinke, C. M., & Derrick, R. M. (2018). An exploration of the role of adverse childhood experiences (ACEs) on youth engagement in residential treatment. *Children and Youth Services Review*, *89*, 355–363. doi: 10.1016/j.childyouth.2018.04.039.

Stout, M. A. (2012). *Native American boarding schools*. Santa Barbara, CA: Greenwood.

Szasz, T. (1961). *The myth of mental illness: Foundations of a theory of personal conduct*. New York: Harper.

Tarren-Sweeney, M. (2007). The Assessment Checklist for Children—ACC: A behavioral rating scale for children in foster, kinship and residential care. *Children and Youth Services Review*, *29*, 672–691. doi: 10.1016/j.childyouth.2007.01.008.

Trent, J. W. (2016). *Inventing the feeble mind: A history of intellectual disability in the United States* (2nd ed.). New York: Oxford University Press.

van IJzendoorn, M. H., Palacios, J., Sonuga-Barke, E. J. S., Gunnar, M. R., Vorria, P., McCall, R. B., Le Mare, L., Bakermans-Kranenburg, M., Dobrova-Krol, N. A., & Juffer, F. (2011). Children in institutional care: Delayed development and resilience. In R. B. McCall, M. H. van IJzendoorn, F. Juffer, C. J. Groark, & Groza, V. K. (Eds.). Children without permanent parents: Research, practice, and policy. *Monographs of the Society for Research in Child Development*, *76*(4), 8–30. doi: 10.1111/j.1540-5834.2011.00626.x.

Webster, R. D., Wente, J., Parris, S. R., & Rus, A. V. (2017). Congregate care settings in the United States. In A. V. Rus, S. R. Parris, & E. Stativa (Eds.), *Child maltreatment in residential care: History, research, and current practice* (pp. 461–475). Cham: Springer.

Weiser, B. (2020, February 21). Beatings, burns and betrayal: The Willowbrook scandal's legacy. *New York Times*, A1.

Whittaker, J. K., Holmes, L., del Valle, J. F., Ainsworth, F., Andreassen, T., Anglin, J., … Zeira, A. (2016). Therapeutic residential care for children and youth: A consensus statement of the International Work Group on Therapeutic Care. *Residential Treatment for Children & Youth*, *33*, 89–106. doi: 10.1080/0886571X.2016.1215755.

Whittaker, J. K., Holmes, L., del Valle, J. F., & James, S. (Eds.). (2023). *Revitalizing residential care for children and youth: Cross-national trends and challenges*. New York: Oxford University Press.

Wilhelm, P. A. (2002). Permanency at what cost?: Five years of imprudence under the Adoption and Safe Families Act of 1997. *Notre Dame Journal of Law, Ethics and Public Policy*, *16*(2), Article 15. Retrieved from: https://scholarship.law.nd.edu/ndjlepp/vol16/iss2/15.

Witmer, L. (1907/1996). Clinical psychology. *The Psychological Clinic*, *1*, 1–9. Reprinted in *American Psychologist*, *51*, 248–251. doi: 10.1037/0003-066X.51.3.248.

Woolford, A. (2015). *This benevolent experiment: Indigenous boarding school, genocide, and redress in Canada and the United States*. Lincoln: University of Nebraska Press.

Zeanah, C. H., Smyke, A. T., & Settles, L. D. (2006). Orphanages as a developmental context for early childhood. In K. McCartney & D. Phillips (Eds.), *Blackwell handbook of early childhood development* (pp. 424–454). Malden, MA: Blackwell. doi: 10.1002/9780470757703.

4 What Explains the Hostility toward Residential Care?

Children and youth have two essential needs. They need stable rearing conditions, ones that they can count on without significant changes in circumstances over time. And they need resources, material and psychological. Stability and resources are most often provided by two parents who give time and emotional support to their children. In situations where this is not possible, it is best for children to be in circumstances that most closely imitate a stable family. This can be an adoptive family, foster care with relatives, or foster care. The thesis of this book is that there are situations when adoption has not occurred or has not worked, and foster care has not worked. When that happens, high-quality residential care can provide the stability and resources that will enhance development (Thoburn, 2023). Often, the residential care can lead to adoption, quality foster care, or reunion with a family of origin. Sometimes the stay in residential care can be short, sometimes months or years, or, rarely, through early adult preparation for independence. However, increasingly, many scholars, professionals, professional organizations, and foundations have argued, vociferously, that children and youth should *never* be placed in residential care except as a one- or two-week stopgap. If residential care is not an option, children and youth may be placed in yet another dysfunctional foster care situation, perhaps one that takes in so many children that it functions like residential care but without the resources or accountability of a children's home or residential treatment center.

Why is there such hostility toward residential care? The common answer is some form of "Research shows..." or "We all know...." In this chapter, we will look at the general nature of the hostility to residential care as it appears in the late 20th and early 21st century writing on residential care. Then we will look in depth at four examples of research that have formed much of the base for the modern critique of residential care. Does research show that residential care is harmful to all children and youth, regardless of age and circumstance? Just how solid is the research base for prohibitions against residential care? This chapter does not review every critique of residential care. However, the instances reviewed are representative and the analysis of these critiques will provide a sketch of the nature of the hostility toward residential care and the research upon which it is based. I note from the start that

DOI: 10.4324/9781003435709-4

these four clumps of research are not independent. The names of some of the researchers in this area appear repeatedly in reports and policy statements. To the degree that their findings and policy statements accurately reflect the dangers of extreme deprivation on infants and young children, their persistence is laudable. To the extent that their findings have been generalized inappropriately across ages, cultures, and sites, the lack of independence is troublesome.

The Nature of the Hostility

The placement of children or youth in residential care commonly referred to as an "institution," "orphanage," or "home" is usually a response to a crisis. Some form of disaster befalls a family, resulting in an inability of surviving members of the family to care for the children or youth. The disasters may be medical, economic, or criminal. In America during the 19th and early 20th centuries, institutions run by private charities built large buildings to house children and youth whose parents had died, or whose single surviving parent could not adequately provide for the child. Child-to-caretaker ratios were large, and children and youth provided much of the labor, including farming, laundry services, and meal preparation. Problems in specific institutions documented in popular literature, news media, and some scholarly reports illustrate egregious conditions and treatment of residents. McKenzie's (1997, 2003) work suggests that more typical orphanages provided good care. However, by the latter third of the 20th century, large institutions as described in the popular literature had all but disappeared in the United States, Canada, and the United Kingdom while they were increasing in number in some developing countries. Both large institutions and residential care that does not resemble the large institutions are seen by many to reflect the same problems as the large orphanages. There is now federal legislation in the United States (The Family First Prevention Services Act of 2018) and professional pronouncements around the world (e.g., from the Annie E. Casey Foundation, the United Nations General Assembly Resolution on the Promotion and Protection of the Rights of Children; the Orthopsychiatric Association; the Lancet Group Commission; the latter two will be analyzed in detail below) that no form of long-term or moderate-term residential care should be funded or licensed anywhere.

Anglin and Knorth (2004) point out that it was not too long ago that residential care was a recognized part of the arsenal of interventions that child welfare workers could selectively use to deal with children and youth who could not live with their families of origin, because they no longer existed, were criminally abusive or neglectful, or involved their children in crimes. Anglin and Knorth cited the declaration from a 1986 conference in Malmö, Sweden, which indicated that community (residential) care had developed to the point where it should be considered an "important available intervention to be used at an appropriate time in the development of those children for whom it is desirable" (p. 142). Less than 20 years later, in the Stockholm Declaration (*Stockholm Declaration on Children and Residential Care*, May, 2003), any sort of residential care was seen as "institutional" and intrinsically damaging, to be used only as a last resort. Anglin and Knorth raised the questions of whether there were no longer children and youth "...being bounced through 10, 20, or even in excess of 30 foster homes?" (p. 142) and asked: what evidence had appeared between the two conference statements that led to the conclusion that residential care was intrinsically evil? I believe the evidence being used, or misused, is what I summarize below.

Throughout the child welfare research literature, the harm caused by residential care is simply assumed. Here is a sampling:

> There is indisputable evidence that institutional care has negative consequences for both individual children and for society at large.
>
> (*Stockholm Declaration on Children and Residential Care*, May, 2003)

> We now know that an institution [residential care] is never the best option for any child.
>
> (Boone, 1999, as cited in Anglin & Knorth, 2004)

> Currently, placement outside the home, particularly in group care, is widely viewed as representing a failure of the system (usually, child welfare), rather than as the targeted use of one of a continuum of legitimate intervention options that can enhance a young person's life situation and, perhaps that of his or her family.
>
> (Beker, 2001, pp. 443–444)

> Child welfare theorists and practice experts in the United States have coalesced around the *philosophical conclusion* that when children cannot remain safely at home they should be placed in family settings whenever possible...
>
> (Alpert & Meezan, 2012, my emphasis)

> ...research consistently chronicles adverse effects of institutional rearing on children's development, particularly in the social-emotional domain.
>
> (Oliveira, Fearon, Belsky, Fachada, & Soares, 2015, p. 161)

> ...fifty years of research reconfirms the same findings: long-term institutionalization in childhoods leads to recurrent problems in interpersonal relationships, a higher rate of personality disorders, and severe parenting difficulties late in life.
>
> (McKenzie, 1997, quoting from Ford and Kroll's, 1995 report from the North American Council on Adoptable Children, p. 5)

Similar statements can be found in a host of reports, article introductions, qualitative reviews, websites, and media articles. Note, the term "institution" is frequently used, but no distinctions are made among institutions, therapeutic residential care, children's homes, and group homes. Just what is the evidence that shows the failures of residential care and led to a very rapid decline in the status of even the best residential care? Is the evidence "philosophical," anecdotal, or based on empirical data? Advocates of residential care "...start out on the defensive, and to advocate for residential care is to make oneself vulnerable to the charge that his or her values are somehow outdated and/or otherwise flawed" (Beker, 2001, p. 444). Should they? Are all or any of the above statements true?

Before we look at specific examples of evidence being used to provide support for the hostility, there are some general problems with residential care, each of which contains at least a grain of legitimacy. First, residential care is expensive. More expensive than adoption or foster care (James, 2011; James, Alemi, & Zepeda, 2013; McCrae, Lee, Barth, & Rauktis, 2010). Although some defenders of residential care have argued that properly calculated, the long-term costs of residential care are lower (Beker, 2001), it seems likely that high-quality residential care will be expensive, at least as measured by short-term outcomes. Second, some claim that residence in group care stigmatizes children or youth within certain cultures (An, Lee, & Chung, 2020; Calheiros, Garrido, Lopes, & Patricio, 2015). Third, being with peers who behave badly may lead to imitative behavior (Osei & Gorey, 2019). Fourth, there is potential in group settings for abuse by staff members and other residents (Moore, McArthur, Death, Tilbury, & Roche, 2017, 2018). Fifth, some argue that instability of staff is endemic to residential care (Hyde & Kammerer, 2009; Palmer, Ahn, Traube, Prindle, & Putnam-Hornstein, 2020). Finally, and perhaps most important, there are concerns that residential care is ineffective or even psychologically damaging (James, 2011; James et al., 2013). Our examination of the research literature in this chapter and the next will call each of these assertions into question.

Examples of the Research Base for Hostility

Included in this critical review are: (a) the single most impactful program of research in residential care, the Bucharest Early Intervention Project; (b) two influential organizational consensus statements that purport to be based on empirical research showing that all residential care is inherently harmful for children of all ages and therefore should be discontinued, one from the Orthopsychiatric Association and one from a Lancet Commission; and (c) a review of research aimed at demonstrating the negative influence of residential care.

Exhibit 1: The impact of the Bucharest Early Intervention Project (BEIP). The Bucharest Early Intervention Project (Nelson, Fox, & Zeanah, 2014) has a special status in the literature on residential care. I agree with Neagu (2021) that the research of the Bucharest Early Intervention Project group has had a strong influence on general statements about residential care by governments, agencies, nongovernment organizations, and the thinking around the United Nations Guidelines for the Alternative Care of Children. The Bucharest project and resulting statements have influenced the view of all types of residential care around the world. The Bucharest Early Intervention Project is directed and staffed by prestigious researchers, and it provides a direct randomized clinical trial of residential (institutional) care compared to foster care. The most readable summary of the Bucharest Early Intervention Project story is the Nelson et al. (2014) book. The technical articles from the project are in dozens of journals. An accessible recent overview is Wade et al. (2022). Technical reports from the age 12 follow-up of the original study are also available (Almas, Degnan, Nelson, Zeanah, & Fox, 2016; Humphreys et al., 2016). A fresh perspective from an insider/outsider is Neagu (2021), a book with interesting new data and much wisdom.

With the fall of the communist regime in Romania in 1989, all kinds of social practices in Romania were opened to scrutiny, including the use of "orphanages." A close examination of the social and political roots of the Romanian institutions for children is beyond the scope of this review. In brief, there had been a concerted effort by the communist government to encourage women to have many children, and, if they were burdensome due to housing or poverty, to hand them over to the state to be raised. The presumption was that the state would do a better job of raising children than parents anyway. There were few true orphans in the institutions. Almost all the children had parents who knew where they were and usually had some contact with them (Neagu, 2021). What stunned the world, starting in the early 1990s, were the pictures of the facilities where large numbers of infants and very young children were housed with high adult-child ratios, little interaction with caregivers, and no toys or books. As told by Nelson et al. (2014), in 2000, a group of American cognitive developmental neuroscientists who had been doing animal research on brain development was given the opportunity to design a study in Romania.

The study the Bucharest Early Intervention Project group designed had a unique and salient feature. After obtaining a sample of children from five institutions and screening them for health and other issues, the children were randomly assigned to remain in the institution or move into foster homes parented by individuals selected by and trained by the Bucharest Early Intervention Project staff. The Bucharest Early Intervention Project became the first and only randomized clinical trial with young children comparing depriving institutional care with a form of family care. Although generalization (external) validity issues remained because neither the institutions nor the children were randomly selected, the research design provided good internal validity (i.e., random assignment ensured that the groups were equivalent to start; see Chapter 3). That allowed for making causal inferences about the effects of deprivation on development. Of course, of particular interest to the cognitive neuroscientists were questions about the amount and timing of experiences on brain development. The researchers were cognizant of the ethical issues involved in the project and obtained advice and approval from various groups (but that did not stop critics from debating additional ethical questions—see Wassenaar, 2006; Zeanah, Fox, & Nelson, 2012). For additional comparison purposes (particularly important because many of the measures, especially those of brain functioning, were not normed for a Romanian population), a community group of local Romanian children who had never been institutionalized was recruited and assessed.

The study included a wide variety of dependent measures that were variously administered at baseline, when participants were six to 30 months of age, prior to the entry of the foster care group to their new homes, and then at ages 30 months, 42 months, 54 months, eight years, and 12 years. They included measures of general cognition (age-appropriate intelligence tests), language, executive functioning, brain imagery, emotional reactivity, attachment, growth, and a measure of epigenetic health (telomere length—shorter lengths are associated with degenerative disease).

The details of the study's results are complex, but the overall patterns are clear. Before the foster care group members left the institution, all the institutionalized children performed below the community comparison group across measures. At each of the subsequent assessment points, the fostered children did better than those left in the institution (those who were in the group called "care as usual"—some of the children who were in the institutionalized group left during the study to be fostered or to be with their biological families, some returning off and on to the institution) on general cognition, language, brain activity, emotional responsiveness, and indicators of attachment. That was not true for measures of executive functioning or gray matter. On most measures, the fostered children did not attain levels equivalent to the community group. At age 12, the mean IQ scores for the fostered group was 23 points lower than the community sample but seven points higher than those who had remained in one of the institutions, Almas et al. (2016). Fostered children did match the community group on emotional responsiveness. On some measures, the difference between the formerly institutionalized and the institutionalized groups was greater when the children had left the institution earlier. At age 12, children who had ever been institutionalized had more reported internalizing and externalizing problems and those who had been fostered had fewer reported externalizing problems than the care as usual group. An interesting finding from the age 12 assessment was that disruption in foster care placement (number of movements among placements) was correlated with the number of externalizing and internalizing problems.

As a research study, the Bucharest Early Intervention Project has several important strengths. A broad range of measures was used, including indicators of physical, psychological, and social development. The study's participants have been followed longitudinally. Perhaps most important, because of the use of random assignment to remain in the institution or to be fostered, causal inferences about the effects of like environments on infants and young children like the ones studied are warranted. That part of the investigation has *internal validity*. The problem is that such inferences have been made, not just for infants and young children like those studied developing in environments like those extremely stark institutions in Romania, but for older children and youth in a wide variety of forms of residential care across the world. The Romanian sample has many unique features that preclude generalization. Most of the infants had been voluntarily given up by their parents for unknown reasons. It is difficult to see just what other identifiable groups are similar enough to the members of the group in its background and experiences to allow for generalization. Generalization of findings from the Bucharest Early Intervention Project to care for older children or even infants and young children in very different environments is a clear violation of the basic principles of *external validity* discussed in Chapter 3. Appropriate generalization of the findings of the Bucharest Early Intervention Project would require replication of the study with older children and youth in residential environments very different than those found in Romania in the 1990s. Yet in a recent summary of the Bucharest Early Intervention Project's longitudinal research, Wade et al. (2022) conclude:

> If there is a single most important legacy to our work, it is to underscore the *urgent need to end institutional rearing and promote high-quality and stable family placements*, along with evidence-based interventions that target the key mechanisms of risk and recovery for neglected young children throughout the world.
>
> (p. 162, my emphasis)

No attempt is made to consider anything but the stark contrast of "institution" versus "family." References to the Bucharest Early Intervention Project are made in scores of journal articles and policy statements without qualification (see the next two exhibits as examples). The Nelson et al. book itself has been cited nearly 400 times according to Google Scholar, most often in reference to groups of children and types of care completely unlike that described in the book.

Exhibit 2: A Consensus Statement endorsed by the Board of Directors of the American Orthopsychiatric Association. In the mid-2010s, The Annie E. Casey Foundation and the Youth Law Center asked a group of child development experts, mostly psychologists, to come together to address the question of how residential care experiences influence children and youth. The aim was to integrate child development research into child welfare policy and practice around the issue of the appropriate role of group care in protecting vulnerable children and adolescents. The members of the group were influential researchers in developmental psychology research, especially infant attachment research. Some had been involved in the Bucharest Early Intervention Project. The statement they developed was approved by the Board of Directors of the American Orthopsychiatric Association (since renamed the Global Alliance for Behavioral Health and Social Justice) and published in their journal in 2014 (Dozier et al., 2014). The association, popularly known as "Ortho" is a multi-disciplinary organization that is usually a secondary professional affiliation for its members. Members come from a wide variety of disciplines, including psychiatry, psychology, social work, law, public health, and many others. Under the general purpose of protecting human rights and preventing mental disorders, Ortho members aim to influence public policy using research-based knowledge about development, families, schools, and community mental health.

The statement is brief (Dozier et al., 2014, p. 219), but it is supplemented by summaries of research for each of ten supporting issues. The statement begins with a sentence that is difficult to challenge: "Every child has a basic right and need to grow up in a safe home with a stable continuous relationship with at least one adult who is a trusted, committed parent figure." There are no conditional statements as to why this does not happen for many children and youth. The second sentence of the statement is direct: "Group settings should not be used as living arrangements, because of their *inherently detrimental effects* on the healthy development of children, regardless of age" (my emphasis added). The statement goes on to state that group care should only be used "when it is the least detrimental alternative" and should "end when it ceases to be the least detrimental alternative for that child."

In their introduction, the Ortho authors note that the United Nations General Assembly in 2010 called for the elimination of large residential care facilities. They state: "We assert a stronger position by contending that institutional care is nonoptimal for children of all ages, including teenagers, and that even smaller care settings can be detrimental to the growth and well-being of youth" (p. 220). The "can be" in that otherwise strong, confident statement provides a convenient out. Nevertheless, the strength and confidence of that statement should be judged against the strength of and confidence in the evidence they provide for their assertions. It is a main thesis of this book that this statement is an inappropriate and unwarranted overgeneralization not backed by the available evidence. I will reserve further comments on the overall statement until we describe each subsidiary point and comment on its research support.

1 **Healthy attachments with a parent figure are necessary for children at all ages and help to reduce problem behaviors and interpersonal difficulties.** Attachment theory, as developed by Bowlby, Ainsworth, Sroufe and a number of the authors of the Ortho statement, figures prominently in the rationale for the statement. Attachment theory emphasizes a healthy infant-adult relationship in which infants emit signals indicating their physical and emotional needs, and adults respond sensitively to those

signals. Over the first year of life, if the system is working, the child develops a sense of efficacy and uses the relationship (or relationships—attachments occur to multiple caregivers) as a secure base for safely exploring the physical and social environment. The development of a secure attachment relies on the availability of a stable, consistent adult figure. A secure attachment bodes well for the subsequent development of cognitive and social-emotional competence. When an attachment figure is not available, youth may become attached to peers who may not provide the resources offered by caring adults and may learn unhealthy, risky behaviors from peers or be abused by peers.

The use of the term "parent figure" is ambiguous. The Ortho authors imply that the parent figure is someone for whom the child has developed an attachment. There is little doubt that a secure attachment acquired in the first two years of life is a good base for healthy development. However, a substantial proportion of children who are in seemingly stable environments do not establish secure attachments. Many, if not most, of the children and youth who find their way to a residential setting never had established a secure relationship with any adult. After many failed foster care home placements, a residential care facility may provide the most consistent, responsive, and stable environment they have ever had (Anglin, 2004). The concerns raised by the authors about peers being a bad influence (iatrogenic effects) rely too much on a laboratory research program (Dishion, McCord, & Poulin, 1999) that has been seriously questioned by researchers studying real-world groups. Weiss, Caron, Ball, Tapp, Johnson and Weisz (2005) found no evidence for iatrogenic effects in their analysis of the laboratory research and a meta-analysis of other studies. In a Teaching Family Model (Boys Town) environment, Lee and Thompson (2009) found that fewer than 10% of the youth in care showed an increase in problem behaviors while in care and that positive peer behaviors inhibited acting out. It is odd that the Ortho group did not cite the Weiss et al. or Lee and Thompson work given that both papers were published in prestigious journals years before the statement was developed.

2 **Especially during adolescence, it is critical to balance children's need for parental control and regulation with their developing needs for autonomy.** The research included in support of this subsidiary statement describes the ideal parent who adjusts control consistent with the child's general developmental needs for autonomy and individual and situational differences. In young children, this occurs in secure attachments where the signal-response system is working well. In a responsive system, adults tailor rules and consequences to the child's needs. For older children and adolescents, the adult needs to know the individual well and be willing and able to adjust controls. "An institutional setting with fixed rules and procedures that are not adapted to the individual is not conducive to the healthy development of autonomy" (p. 221).

The standard of parenting described here is high for even the most well-adjusted families in the best of circumstances. No research is cited to indicate that this kind of parenting is normative *anywhere*. One of the defining characteristics of the group of children and youth in the child welfare system is a history of being cared for by adults who have not handled the autonomy/control balance well. The real issue here is the quality of care, regardless of who is providing it (see Chapter 5). The statement about the inflexibility of group care is based on presumption, or a stereotype of group care, not research. No evidence is cited to support it.

3 **Child-sensitive exercise of authority is critical to healthy development.** The support for this subordinate statement relies heavily on the work of one of the authors of the consensus (Smetana). The argument is that children, especially adolescents, are in ongoing negotiations about parental regulation. While they accept parental authority in the domains of morality, societal conventions, and health and safety, adolescents do not accept regulation in personal domains such as physical appearance, privacy, choice of friends, and leisure activities. Parents must balance regulation and monitoring with autonomy in a close, trusting relationship. In residential settings, adults are likely to overregulate in the personal domain and are unlikely to develop a trusting, responsive relationship.

Again, the parenting standard set is quite high, and no normative data are cited. The youth in residential care rarely have experienced such well-titrated regulation in their families. There probably are more rules in most group care, but if the care is of high quality, trusting, responsive relationships do develop (see Chapters 6 and 7) and flexibility may be greater than in the individual's family of origin or the multiple foster care settings they typically have experienced.

4 **Group care is not an appropriate living arrangement, and it can never substitute for a home environment.** Although this claim suggests a conclusion, it is used as an out for short-term stays in setting such as wilderness camps or psychiatric facilities (therapeutic residential care). These time-limited settings provide opportunities for engaged relationships with adults who act as attachment figures before they go home. In contrast, in group care, youth rely on a constantly rotating staff to provide guidance and support.

This assertion seems to be aimed at long-term residential care for adolescents. The use of "never" and "not appropriate" calls for better research support and the use of "attachment figure" is odd given that we know that attachment formation requires months or years according to traditional attachment theory (e.g., Ainsworth, Blehar, Waters, & Wall, 1978). Once again, the assumption of "constantly rotating staff" is a characteristic attributed to group care without supporting evidence.

5 **Group care itself may be related to an increased likelihood of problem behavior.** This contention is supported by the same research on iatrogenic effects cited in support of Statement #1. An additional non-equivalent control

group study (Ryan, Marshall, Herz, & Hernandez, 2008) is cited to support the notion that those who have been in residential care are more likely to be arrested. Also, "...group care prevents children having access to peers who are coping well with everyday life, who do not have behavioral or emotional problems, and who can provide positive peer support" (p. 221).

The last sentence does not cite any evidence. It assumes that all children in residential care are isolated from competent peers. That is demonstrably untrue in most cases. For example, residents in many children's homes and group homes attend community schools, recreation centers, and churches. The "may be" qualification in the statement is appropriate given the weakness of the research. The Ryan et al. study tries to control for group differences statistically, but ultimately cannot pull off any valid cause-effect inferences (see the discussion of this study in Chapter 3).

6 **Group care may cause psychological harm even in typically developing children.** The Ortho authors use the natural experiment of the Israeli kibbutzim as a "semi-institutional" analogy to residential care to support this claim. They say longitudinal research on the children of the kibbutz suggests that even children who had not experienced prior trauma show problems with attachment security when they are subjected to group sleeping arrangements. They argue, however, that some parents personalized the bedtime experience of their children and violated kibbutz rules, thus buffering their children from the negative effects of unnatural group sleeping arrangements.

This subsidiary statement is remarkably broad. Yet no basis for generalizing from the kibbutz to any modern instantiation of residential care is provided. Perhaps the authors are considering the sleeping arrangements for infants in the extremely deprived environments of Romanian orphans and the like. Regardless, the description of parents who broke the rules of the kibbutzim is not analogous of the parenting experience of the typical child or youth in residential care. In direct contradiction to this statement, Macarov (2008) argues that on the whole, the kibbutzim experience provides support for the efficacy of group care.

7 **Group care for abused and maltreated children also may be physically dangerous.** "There are several highly publicized cases of the physical and sexual abuse of children in various countries..." (p. 222). One of the authors is a co-author of papers showing that self-reported and caregiver-reported physical and sexual abuse is higher in foster care and residential settings than in families in the general population (Euser, Alink, Tharner, van IJzendoorn, & Bakermans-Kraneburg, 2013, 2014). This may be due to instability in caregivers, high staff turnover, or the instability of groups of residents. The authors conclude: "Exposing vulnerable children to increased risk for maltreatment in an intervention administered because of maltreatment is unjustified" (p. 222).

The last statement is inarguable. Bad childcare is bad childcare, whether it is administered in residential care, foster care, or families of origin (recent "highly publicized cases" concerning the main alternative to residential care, family foster care, are instructive; e.g., https://www.usatoday.com/in-depth/news/investigations/2021/03/18/foster-care-children-starved-beaten-molested-florida-reports-show/6782615002/). Abuse is a sign of inadequate quality of care. Safeguards are needed wherever children and youth live. However, there are good reasons to consider the "may be" of the statement. If care is of high quality and includes proper monitoring, there is no reason to see it as inherently more dangerous than any other care setting, including families. In his historical overview, Jones (1993) argues that even the early 20th century orphanages were "...remarkably free of scandals involving child abuse or neglect" (p. 471). After a careful analysis of child protection services records in the United Kingdom, Gallagher (2000) concludes that institutional sexual abuse was uncommon and:

> Contrary to media representations, the institutional abuse reported here was not just a problem of children's homes, social work or the public sector, but occurred in a wide variety of settings and sectors and was perpetrated by a range of occupational groups.
>
> (p. 795)

Mark Smith (2010) argues that we should be careful about generalizations from "highly publicized cases." Although the idea that historic care settings were characterized by "endemic abuse and systematic cover-up" has become "...the default position of social work academics" (p. 304), Smith argues that the documentary evidence of widespread abuse is often hard to find. He analyzes the work of the Scottish Government's *Systemic Review of Historical Abuse 2000*s. Smith points out that a helpline set up to advise victims of residential care abuse had to be closed when it received only one call in a three-month period. Obviously, no matter how rare or widespread abuse is, it needs to be addressed each time wherever it occurs.

8 **There is no demonstrable therapeutic necessity for group care to be used as a long-term living arrangement.** Substance abuse, sexual acting out behavior, and delinquency can better be treated in communities rather than in residential settings. Multisystem forms of therapy and foster care do not require residence and work better closer to the family setting. "Group care should be reserved for use when it is the least detrimental alternative for children and adolescents" (p. 222).

Although the assertion that children and youth are better served in their homes and communities is contentious, I will not argue the point. I hope that turns out to be correct. However, problems centered in the child are not what leads to much residential care. Instead, the problems are in the community, the family of origin, or the foster care system. The latter has often been worked to exhaustion with placements for individual children numbered upwards sometimes to the dozens. It is for the latter group that residential care can provide the stability and resources that are truly therapeutic (e.g., Calheiros, Silva, & Patrício, 2020).

9 **Even children who have never experienced secure attachments can develop them in appropriate family settings.** Adolescents, even ones whose developmental journeys have been difficult, can form secure attachments to foster caregivers. The likelihood of such attachments is associated with the quality of the interactions with the foster parent.

 Of course, this is good news. If high-quality foster parents were consistently available, there would be fewer failed placements. In an ideal world, every child and youth would be placed in such a situation. The high median number of foster placements per foster child indicates we do not live in that world (e.g., Biehal, 2007; Rock, Michelson, Thomson, & Day, 2015). Older children and youth are much harder to place and much less likely to be adopted out of foster care. In high-quality residential care where caregivers stay for months or years, those same attachments can form.

10 **Group care should never be used for young children.** Much data from the 1990s and 2000s from eastern European and Chinese institutions show that infants who are not fostered or adopted into families have cognitive and social-emotional difficulties. Ones who are, can make remarkable progress.

 Indeed, the literature on infants and young children raised in extremely deprived environments indicates they do not do well. Unfortunately, we know little about the effects of higher quality residential experiences. Based on what we know about early cognitive development and attachment (e.g., Bilson & Bywaters, 2020), along with the most basic complexities of raising infants, I think it may be safe to say that this statement holds even for less deprived environments. However, there is much evidence that the brains of infants are quite resilient (e.g., Pignotti, 2011; Wastell & White, 2012). The thousands of infants around the world who cannot be cared for in optimal environments should not be seen as lost causes as a result. Fortunately, in the United States and other well-off countries, it is infants and young children who are most easily fostered into stable families and who are most likely to be subsequently adopted (Foster Care Statistics 2019 (childwelfare.gov)).

General comments on the Orthopsychiatric consensus. This "consensus" has had broad influence. It is frequently cited as evidence that there is no need to consider residential care as anything but an unattractive last resort for children of any age or circumstance. For example, in a Brookings Institution report on foster care, Haskins (2017, pp. 3–4) refers to the Ortho consensus, stating:

> There is now almost universal agreement that group or institutional care should be considered an option of last resort. In 2014, a group of ten leading child welfare researchers with extensive careers of research

> on children felt so strongly about this issue that they issued a "consensus statement" on group care. Their conclusion, stated with admirable conciseness, is that children should be placed in group care only "when necessary therapeutic mental health services cannot be delivered in a less restrictive setting."

There are numerous reasons why there should be no universal agreement based on Dozier et al. (2014). First, it is the nature of social science research that findings are rarely absolutely stated. There is usually considerable room for doubt. Such doubt is reflected in the "may be's" and "can's" of sub-statements 5, 6, 7, 9. The other subsidiary statements are more strongly stated. That certainty is much too strong for the research bases provided (and available). Because the term "group care" is used so broadly, it includes almost any care outside of families of origin, adoptive families, and foster families. The research cited is much more limited. The "group care" in the best available literature is from the extremely deprived orphanages of eastern Europe and Asia. Almost none of the studies cited by Dozier et al. have been conducted in the United States, Canada, the United Kingdom, or continental Western Europe where children are rarely exposed to such stark conditions (even the laxest license requirements would disallow anything like the horrific conditions where the children in the extant studies resided). There are too many sample, methodological, and measurement limitations in much of the research to allow absolutist conclusions such as those provided in the Ortho consensus.

Second, the strength of the available research is inversely related to age. The infant research, although on a very narrow range of environments, is methodologically stronger. There is almost no literature cited on children over age 5 and the literature cited on adolescence is frequently on laboratory studies, not on youth in care. The research on infants and very young children has been inappropriately generalized across age. Similar overgeneralizations have been made across settings.

Third, the principles underlying the general statement and its subsidiaries would have been very similar if the Ortho group had been asked "What is ideal parenting like?" That standard would be hard for even stable, intact, non-traumatized, well-resourced families to meet. Fourth, there is a strong ivory tower quality to this document. It appears to be written in response to a question like "Based on what we know about child development, what possibly could go wrong in group care?" There seems to be a failure on the part of the group to recognize the reality that there are children for whom the foster care and adoption systems have not worked. Residential care is populated by many young people whose lives have been made chaotic by placement after placement after placement. Another "family" that they know is not their family is of little help (see Proposition 7 in Chapter 8).

Finally, the Ortho group does not adequately deal with the operational meaning of "least detrimental alternative." That would require a much more nuanced statement recognizing individual differences in children and youth, differences in their circumstances, and differences in group care. It would require a balanced assessment of the practical issues of adoption, foster care, and families in serious trouble. It seems undeniable that for some individuals, high-quality (see Chapter 6 on quality) residential care is what will meet their needs for a few months, a few years, or into young adulthood. But that is denied by the Ortho consensus. Categorically condemning residential care is not demanded by the evidence and is not helpful.

Exhibit 3: Statement of Policy from the Lancet Group Commission. The editors of *The Lancet*, perhaps the world's most prestigious medical journal, occasionally commission academic researchers to address pressing issues and make policy recommendations. Two recent publications (Goldman et al., 2020; van IJzendoorn et al., 2020) are part of a commission that strongly condemns all kinds of group care (https://www.thelancet.com/commissions/deinstitutionalisation). Van IJzendoorn et al. (2020) report meta-analyses of hundreds of studies from the previous seven decades and use the Bucharest Early Intervention Project as a comparison. Their analysis provides the foundation for the policies outlined in Goldman et al. (2020), a statement of policy from the Lancet Group Commission. The policies in the latter are bold and go well beyond the available data in calling for a literal cancellation of residential care except for very small homes targeted for special groups. The two papers can be seen as a follow-up to the Bucharest Early Intervention Project. Many of the members of the Bucharest Early Intervention Project group are coauthors on one or both papers. The two articles represent a great deal of effort. The authors of the data-based article briefly review the historical and cultural context of institutionalization, characterize general aspects of institutions, and describe the populations of children served globally. Their third section provides a set of meta-analyses of 308 studies addressing two major questions. First, is growing up in an institution detrimental compared to those who group up in their family of origin, foster care, or were adopted? Second, if a child leaves an institution, does developmental catch-up occur? In addition to comparing the overall differences, the results of the meta-analyses are compared to the findings of the Bucharest Early Intervention Project, the only extant study that involved children randomly assigned to go into foster care versus remaining in an institution (see Exhibit 1). The assumption is that the results of the meta-analyses can be considered more reliable if they are similar to those from the randomized groups of the Bucharest Early Intervention Project with its internal validity.

The results of a series of meta-analyses (the investigators used a sophisticated set of statistical procedures to check for sample bias, quality of study, etc.) provide answers to the two questions. Regarding differences, the investigators find strong effect sizes (i.e., significant statistical differences favoring the non-institutionalized) on measures of growth, head circumference (as a stand-in for brain size), cognitive development, and attention. There are smaller effect sizes for physical health and socio-emotional development. When compared to data from the Bucharest Early Intervention Project, the differences between institutionalized and noninstitutionalized are similar in each domain, except the difference on cognitive development was greater in the Bucharest Early Intervention Project. There are many fewer studies relevant to the question of catch-up. The available results indicate that significant catch-up is evident on measures of growth (21 studies), head circumference (7), and cognition (14), but not socioemotional behavior (11). There are not enough studies to test catch-up on attention. These results are similar in most domains to those from the institutionalized-foster care differences in the Bucharest Early Intervention Project (the foster care group generally did not do as well as the never-institutionalized group). The researchers speculate that their results are likely an underestimation of the detrimental effects of institutionalization for two reasons. In the Bucharest Early Intervention Project, some members of the institutionalized group had entered foster care before all measures were obtained and unique physical and psychological problems caused by institutionalization may not have been picked up by the relatively insensitive measures used in the available studies. The authors anticipated the policies provided in the Goldman et al. paper in their summary:

> Every effort should be made to minimise children's exposure to institutional care. Reducing the number of children entering institutions and increasing the number leaving institutions is urgently needed. Where institutional care is considered absolutely necessary, the length of stays should be as short as possible, even if care is adequate.
>
> [van IJzendoorn et al., 2020, summary, p. 703]

The second Lancet paper (Goldman et al., 2020) offers dozens of recommendations on the international care of children. No new data are provided. The connection to the meta-analysis is basically the simple dichotomy that institutions = bad, family = good. The obvious conclusion is that whatever needs to be done to keep children out of institutions and in families should be done.

What does the Bucharest Early Intervention Project and related work have to say about the kind of residential care offered in the North America, continental Western Europe, and other places in children's homes and therapeutic residential care? The elegance of the Bucharest Early Intervention Project's randomized clinical trial provides solid evidence that extremely depriving environments like those found in Romania in the late 20th century are causally linked to bad developmental outcomes. It shows that those kinds of young children who are removed from that kind of environment and provided with care from sensitive, responsive, adults can make substantial recovery in general cognition and language, and indicators of physical and socioemotional development. As I argue in my comments on Exhibit 1, this research tells us little or nothing about the impact of very different early environments or later environments for older children and youth. As we have seen, that has not stopped some policy makers, including the Lancet Commission, from overgeneralizing the results to all residential care. Again, I find myself agreeing with Neagu (2021): "Using a study carried out in one institution and extending its findings to all group ages and across the globe is generalisation beyond limitation and cannot be scientifically sound" (p. 196). Neagu goes on to say that one of the surprises in her findings was "...the positive accounts of residential care. They suggest that the current policy on deinstitutionalisation is a red herring" (Neagu, 2021, p. 203).

The range of institutions covered in the first Lancet paper is broader than the Bucharest study. However, there are significant limitations to generalizing those results too. Meta-analysis can be a useful tool for summarizing a large research literature if the question involved is clear and the independent variables (experimental and comparison groups) and dependent variables (measurements) are tightly defined. The question here is clear enough, but the independent and dependent variables are a mess. I have already discussed that knowing the independent variable is in this research area is one of the major threats to our understanding of residential care (Chapter 3). The Lancet Commission defines "institutionalization" as follows: "For the purposes of this Commission, we define an institution as a publicly or privately managed and staffed collective living arrangement for children that is not family based" (Goldman et al., 2020, p. 704). Included are orphanages, children's institutions, group homes, infant homes, children's villages, and similar residential settings for children (none of these categories are defined or described) from across the globe. The studies included in the meta-analysis typically used non-experimental designs, unable to take into account pre-existing differences between institutional groups and comparison groups. The meta-analysis combines infants, children, and youth without regard to distinctions. There is no attempt to measure differences in the quality of children's experiences. "Family" is not defined, but clearly whatever it is, it is positive. It appears to me that "family" is being equated with the much more emotionally laden term "home."

In part, the investigators recognize the independent variable problem themselves. They point out that institutions vary greatly in quality on many characteristics, including staff training and turnover, child-to-caregiver ratios, health and nutrition provisions, hygiene standards, and the responsiveness of staff members to residents. They then assert, without evidence, that typically, none of these is adequate in institutions. Interpreting the meaning of the independent variable in the meta-analysis is exacerbated by the range of dates and the sites of the studies used. "Institutionalization" as an independent variable represents studies from a 65-year period, across 68 countries, across many ages (although heavily weighted toward infants and very young children), and many different kinds of "institutionalization."

On the dependent variable side, only very gross indicators are used. Meta-analyses need some basic numbers to work with. The researchers bore down to the most basic means (group averages) and standard deviations (indicators of the dispersion of scores) in the hundreds of studies examined. The dependent variable "cognitive development" is made up of scores of different measures of varying reliability and validity. What does "cognitive development" mean then? It is hard to know. "Socioemotional development" is no clearer except in a supplemental presentation of attachment measurement in infants (using the Ainsworth Strange Situation, a fascinating measure with its own problems of use over time and across parenting cultures). Head circumference has fewer measurement differences across studies, but its meaning is not straightforward. In short, the dependent variables used in the meta-analyses are of unknown construct validity.

The large number of recommendations by the Lancet Commission includes genuinely insightful suggestions about how families can be strengthened. There are common sense recommendations that attack child neglect, abuse, institutional and governmental corruption and for these, we did not need a data base to show us what is right and wrong. Also, there are many recommendations that glibly ignore the complexities of family preservation, foster care, adoption, and family life (just one example from the recommendations, so as to not belabor this: if a child was institutionalized because of parental drug or alcohol addiction, get the parents off the drugs or alcohol while children remain in the home with the assurance from a social worker that they are safe). Also unaddressed are the fiscal, physical, and cultural dimensions of many of the recommendations and actual action agents are not identified.

As far as applying to North American and most Western European residential care, the report is 40–70 years too late. Infants and young children have not been "institutionalized" in the United States and elsewhere for a long time. The authors of van IJzendoorn et al. (2020) note that fact themselves:

> After decades of declining use, institutional care for young children essentially disappeared in the USA after passage of the Adoption Assistance and Child Welfare Act of 1980, which stipulated that children be placed in the least restrictive (most family-like) setting available.
>
> (p. 705)

Of the 34,823 children in institutions involved in the meta-analyses, a total of 290 came from institutions in the United States (<1%). I suspect that most of those 290 were in studies conducted many decades ago. There may be American residences for children and youth that should be closed, but we have known why they should be closed for a long time. That has not and will not keep people from generalizing the results to good residential care for older children and youth. And that is a problem.

Exhibit 4: "Child violence experiences in institutionalised/orphanage care": A review of reviews. Sherr, Roberts, and Gandhi (2017) is a review of studies of potentially bad outcomes in residential care. It includes a review of two previous reviews (Johnson Browne & Hamilton-Giachritsis, 2006; van IJzendoorn, Luijk, & Juffer, 2008). If there is a substantial research base of support for the hostility toward residential care, this should be a good place to find it. Although the title of the paper says it is about child violence experiences, Sherr et al. broaden the meaning of violence (and abuse) to include cognitive and social-emotional damage to children and youth in care. The review focuses on: (a) how prevalent violent behavior, staff/adult toward child and peer to peer, is in institutions; (b) what interventions have been shown to reduce violence; and (c) how common violence, as indicated by neglect, leads to problems in cognitive and social-emotional development.

The researchers identified nine studies on the prevalence of **violent behavior**, all from the early 2010s and including children and youth from seven to 20 years of age. Three studies come from Tanzania, two from Romania, and one each from Kazakhstan, Netherlands, and Israel and one involves institutions from five Asian and African countries. The authors conclude: "The limited data suggest a pervasive abuse problem for children in institutions, however abuse was defined. When comparisons are available (4 studies) the levels were higher than other forms of care or general population rates" (p. 41).

The self-reports used in these studies indicate unacceptably high rates of violence from staff members at the institutions sampled. The Netherlands data (Euser et al., 2014) are clearest because of its national sample. The usual problem of detailing the nature of the independent variable in this area of research is exacerbated here by the wide range of cultures involved. It is particularly problematic that there are no studies from anglophone countries or Northern Europe. Along with many others, I argue, the central issue about the effects of residential care is the quality of care. We know little about the quality of care in the institutions studied here.

The authors found only three studies on the **reduction of abuse** of adolescent residents, two from Tanzania and one from Portugal. The studies reported dramatic decreases in abusive behavior by staff after interventions. The dramatic decreases in abuse after intervention suggest that staff training originally must not have been very extensive, further suggesting that the quality of care is suspect. It is encouraging to find that staff behavior can be modified relatively easily (see the Duke Positive Outcomes for Orphans studies reviewed in Chapter 5).

The focus of the Sherr et al. review shifts when they consider the effect of deprived environments on cognitive and social-emotional behavior. They first briefly summarize the findings from two earlier reviews of the "effect" of institutionalization on behavior. In the first of the earlier reviews, Johnson et al. (2006) review 27 relevant studies from 1944 to 2006. Twelve of the studies measured attachment behavior in some form. In 11 of the 12, institutionalization was associated with difficulties in attachment. Seventeen of the studies measured some form of social behavior. Sixteen of the 17 showed some problem in social behavior. Thirteen of the studies included measures of cognitive development. All but one reported cognitive deficits associated with institutionalization. Johnson et al. indicate that the degree of deficit experienced correlates with the standard of care.

All the studies in Johnson et al. are on children who had been in institutions during infancy or early childhood. Only two were conducted in this century. The 12 studies on attachment include three in which there is no description of the institutions, two from the United Kingdom and one from United States. Five of the studies are of children in the United Kingdom or Canada who had been adopted from Romanian orphanages that were extremely poor environments; in one case the caregiver to infant ratio ranged from 1:10 to 1:20. The other four studies came from Tizard's research program on children who had been in a children's home in the United Kingdom with relatively high standards (see the discussion of the Tizard studies in Chapter 2). Among the 17 studies that include measures of social behavior, two from the United States provide no description of the institutions involved. Ten are studies of children who had been in orphanages in Romania or eastern Europe. Four come from the Tizard sequence and one was conducted in group homes in a lower-class section of Los Angeles. Four of the 13 studies that include measures of cognitive development provide no description of the institutions, three from the United Kingdom and one from the United States. Four are from Romanian or eastern European orphanages. The four Tizard studies are included as is the one from Los Angeles.

In the second of the previous reviews Sherr et al. report on, van IJzendoorn et al. (2008) identify 42 papers on studies from 19 countries looking at cognitive development of infants and young children in orphanages. They report 75 outcomes from the studies that compare scores to peers reared by their parents or foster parents or to standardized test norms. Most of the children were still infants or young children under six years of age. More than 15 different scales were used to measure cognitive status with an intelligence quotient (IQ; for older children) or developmental quotient (DQ; for infants). No details of any kind on the orphanages are provided in about half the studies. Caregiver to child ratios ranged from 1:2.6 to 1:20 (the latter in a Romanian orphanage). Measures include length of stay in the orphanage, age at assessment, and Human Development Index scores (HDI; a measure combining life expectancy, educational levels, and income for the country the children were from). The results show that children growing up in orphanages had a lower IQ or DQ average than peers or norms. Infants with earlier placements in the orphanage (before two years) had lower scores and so did those in countries with lower HDI scores. Length of stay in the orphanage was not correlated with cognitive scores.

Putting aside the well-known problems of trying to measure intelligence before the age of two, the findings of the van IJzendoorn et al. review support the notion that extremely deprived environments are not good for infants and young children. While in many reviews representation of children from 19 countries would be a positive, here the lack of information on the environments children were living in makes it difficult to identify independent-dependent variable relationships. Of the 42 papers represented, nine were conducted in the United States. The publication dates of those papers are 1945, 1947, 1956, 1958, 1963, 1965, 1966, 1973, and 2002. Caregiver-child ratios ranged from 1:2.6 to 1:8.5. Just what were the environments these infants and young children were living in like? Are they representative of the residential care of their time, let along that available in the 21st century (if indeed, you could find organizations in the United States providing institutional care for infants and young children in 2023)?

After reviewing the previous reviews, Sherr et al. conduct their own. Among the 66 studies Sherr et al. identify, 45 include direct measures of child cognition. Forty-two indicate associated deficits in cognition among those in orphanages whereas only three do not. The latter three, from the Positive Outcomes for Orphans study based at the Duke Global Health Institute will be discussed in the next chapter. Four other studies show indirect evidence of detrimental effects of institutional care on infants and young children. The authors use multiple papers reporting on the outcomes of the Bucharest Early Intervention Project, which consistently find that movement of children from severely deprived orphanages with very high caregiver to infant ratios to family foster care homes leads to cognitive improvements. Of the 66 papers identified, 43 report on effects on social and behavioral development. All but two report detrimental associations. Thus, Sherr et al.'s updated findings support those from Johnson et al. and van IJzendoorn et al.'s.

In their conclusion, Sherr et al. note that causal pathways between orphanages and psychological damage are difficult to sort out because of the inability to randomly assign children (ethically) to conditions. They do not distinguish different types of residential care or differences in the quality of care, nor do they discuss differentiations related to age or country. All the studies on cognitive development were on children who had been in orphanages during infancy and/or early childhood. Two-thirds of the orphanages studied were in Romania, conducted mostly by Michael Rutter's group, or the Bucharest Early Intervention Project group. Most of the other third were on orphanages in Russia, China, Turkey, or other countries in institutions with woefully inadequate resources. None of the studies were of children who had been in residential care in the United Kingdom, the United States, or Canada. A few of the additional studies that included social and behavioral measures but not cognitive measures, did include older children but, again, none were done in the United Kingdom, United States, or Canada and involved very large institutions in Turkey.

Summary: Does Research Show That All Residential Care Is Harmful to Children and Youth?

A quarter century ago, John McCall (1999) wrote a critique of the "orphanage literature." He points out the many methodological problems with the extant literature at the time on the effects of being reared in orphanages. The studies he reviews were almost exclusively on convenience samples of infants and young children or older children who had been in institutions when they were very young (most of which are cited in one or more of the exhibits above). McCall points out that the environments at the orphanages were not observed or described in any detail. The orphanage experienced was assumed, without evidence, to have been sterile and unchallenging whereas home care was assumed to be warm and stimulating. He suggests that the small literature could be characterized as a "clinical search for psychological damage" (p. 147). None of it deals with practical issues of siblings, age in care, vocational training, or a host of other issues. McCall concludes: "Critics of orphanage care seem overzealous to produce negative evidence and then generalize their findings to all orphans or orphanages" (p. 147). A decade after McCall's review, David Macarov (2008), Professor Emeritus of Hebrew University, examined published papers on group care that had appeared in the subsequent period. He found no intervening research that would alter McCall's conclusions (or, likely, the ones here).

Is there "indisputable, overwhelming evidence," of the negative psychological consequences on children and youth who have experienced group care? Based on the available empirical literature, the hostility toward residential care in all countries and all ages (Dozier et al., 2014; Goldman et al., 2020; Stockholm Declaration on Residential Care, 2003) still comes from a severely limited research base. There is a yawning gap between the available data and the negative rhetoric about the detrimental effects of residential care children and youth receive in the United States, United Kingdom, Canada and other well-resourced countries. Macarov (2008), argues that the negative perception of residential care stems from a "quasi-religious" belief that children can only grow up healthy, happy, and competent in a nuclear family. To question that belief is outright subversive. "The possibility of positive effects from growing up in a healthy, nurturing environment in an institution seems to be written off in advance..." (Macarov, 2008, p. 108).

It is clear from the available literature that when infants and young children are raised in extremely deprived environments that they do not develop optimally (The Leiden Conference, 2012). Although the data base for the effects of much more enriched environments for infants is limited (see the St. Petersburg intervention study for a demonstration of the positive effects of enrichment, The St. Petersburg-USA Orphanage Research Team, 2008) there is probably good reason. High-quality care for infants is seen as impractically expensive. Moreover, when it comes to finding adoptive and foster care homes, it is much easier to do so for infants and young children. The problems with foster care (e.g., Chambers et al., 2018) that lead children and youth into residential care, including multiple placements and large sibling groups, are not yet present.

Otherwise, blanket condemnation of residential care based on any available research is simply inappropriate. The single weakest aspect of this research literature is the lack of specification of the pseudo-independent variable (pseudo- in every case but the Bucharest Early Intervention Project). "Institution," "congregate care," "children's home," etc. are used without detail across scores of residences in dozens of countries. The largest portion of the research comes from orphanages in Romania, Russia, India, and Turkey, all places where resources for children needing a home were or are limited. We have reasonably good descriptions of those awful places and even telling photographs of rooms crowded with cribs and benches full of young children with nothing to do. Otherwise, the residential care in published studies could mean anything from small group homes (rarely) to large wards of untended children. Measures of quality of care are largely absent or seen as irrelevant. The other obvious weakness in the literature is the lack of research on older children and adolescents. Perhaps because the data from the literature on children and youth often run counter to the negative perception of residential care (see the next chapter), they do not receive the attention received by the infant studies in deprived environments when policies are formed.

The overgeneralization of findings, across age, environment, culture, and measure is rampant. As a research child psychologist, I am surprised that so many professionals in child welfare have so consistently and confidently condemned all residential care on such flimsy evidence. I suspect that some version of what Lear (1998) calls "knowingness" is at work. Knowingness is the belief that we already know about something. Therefore, there is no need to ask incisive questions, critique current knowledge, reconsider the sources from which knowledge comes, or gather relevant data. Knowingness creates the "conventional" in conventional wisdom. "Research says" (even when it does not). "Everybody knows" (even when they do not). "*I* know" (even when my experience is limited and distorted). This overconfidence exacerbates simplistic beliefs such as "families are always good and residential care is always bad" or "the worst mother is better than the best institution." For over a century, especially in anglophone countries, to be "progressive" has been to advocate the end of residential care. Research on infants and very young children in deprived environments reinforces the knowingness about the "enormous harm" of residential care. In the next chapter, we will consider research that provides a very different picture than that provided by the research on the effects of extreme deprivation on infants.

References

Ainsworth, M. D. S., Blehar, M. C., Waters, E., & Wall, S. (1978). *Patterns of attachment: A psychological study of the strange situation*. Hillsdale, NJ: Erlbaum.

Almas, A. N., Degnan, K. A., Nelson, C. A., Zeanah, C. H., & Fox, N. A. (2016). IQ at age 12 following a history of institutional care: Findings from the Bucharest Early Intervention Project. *Developmental Psychology*, *52*, 1858–1866. doi: 10.1037/dev0000167.

Alpert, L. T., & Meezan, W. (2012). Moving away from congregate care: One state's path to reform and lessons for the field. *Children and Youth Services Review*, *34*, 1519–1532. doi: 10.1016/j.childyouth.2012.04.003.

An, E. M., Lee, S. J., & Chung, I.-J. (2020). The effects of the stigma trajectory of adolescents in out-of-home care on self-esteem and antisocial behavior. *Children and Youth Services Review*, *116*, 105167. doi: 10.1016/j.childyouth.2020.105167.

Anglin, J. P. (2004). Creating "well-functioning" residential care and defining its place in a system of care. *Child & Youth Care Forum*, *33*, 175–192. doi: 10.1023/B:CCAR.0000029689.70611.0f.

Anglin, J. P., & Knorth, E. J. (2004). Competing declarations on residential care for children and youth—Stockholm Versus Malmö [Editorial]. *Child and Youth Care Forum*, *33*, 141–149. doi: 10.1023/B:CCAR.0000029720.18947.66.

Beker, J. (2001). Back to the future: Effective residential group care and treatment for children and youth and the Fritz Redl Legacy. *Child & Youth Care Forum*, *30*, 443–455. doi: 10.1023/A:1015329501206.

Biehal, N. (2007). Reuniting children with their families: Reconsidering the evidence on timing, contact and outcomes. *British Journal of Social Work*, *37*, 807–823. doi: 10.1093/bjsw/bcl051.

Bilson, A., & Bywaters, P. (2020). Born into care: Evidence of a failed state. *Children and Youth Services Review*, *116*, 105164. doi: 10.1016/j.childyouth.2020.105164.

Calheiros, M. M., Garrido, M. V., Lopes, D., & Patrício, J. N. (2015). Social images of residential care: How children, youth and residential care institutions are portrayed? *Children and Youth Services Review*, *55*, 159–169. doi: 10.1016/j.childyouth.2015.06.004.

Calheiros, M. M., Silva, C., & Patrício, J. N. (2020). Maltreatment and youth self-representations in residential care: The moderating role of individual and placement variables. *Children and Youth Services Review*, *116*, 105230. doi: 10.1016/j.childyouth.2020.105230.

Chambers, R. M., Crutchfield, R. M., Willis, T. Y., Cuza, H. A., Otero, A., Goddu Harper, S. G., & Carmichael, H. (2018). "It's just not right to move a kid that many times": A qualitative study of how foster care alumni perceive placement moves. *Children and Youth Services Review*, *86*, 76–83. doi: 10.1016/j.childyouth.2018.01.028.

Dishion, T. J., McCord, J., & Poulin, F. (1999). When interventions harm: Peer groups and problem behavior. *American Psychologist*, *54*, 755–764. doi: 10.1037/0003-066X.54.9.755.

Dozier, M., Kaufman, J., Kobak, R., O'Connor, T. G., Sagi-Schwartz, A., Scott, S, … Zeanah, C. H. (2014). Consensus statement on group care for children and adolescents: A statement of Policy of the American Orthopsychiatric Association. *American Journal of Orthopsychiatry*, *84*, 219–225. doi: 10.1037/ort0000005.

Euser, S., Alink, L. R. A., Tharner, A., van IJzendoorn, M. H., & Bakermans-Kranenburg, M. (2013). The prevalence of child sexual abuse in out-of-home care: A comparison between abuse in residential and in foster care. *Child Maltreatment, 18*, 221–231. doi: 10.1177/1077559513489848.

Euser, S., Alink, L. R. A., Tharner, A., van IJzendoorn, M. H., & Bakermans-Kranenburg, M. (2014). Out of home placement to promote safety?: The prevalence of physical abuse in residential and foster care. *Children and Youth Services Review, 37*, 64–70. doi: 10.1016/j.childyouth.2013.12.002.

Gallagher, B. (2000). The extent and nature of known cases of institutional child sexual abuse. *British Journal of Social Work, 30*, 795–817. doi: 10.1093/bjsw/30.6.795.

Goldman, P. S., Bakermans-Kranenburg, M. J., Bradford, B., Christopoulos, A., Ken, P. L. A., Cuthbert, C., ... Sonuga-Barke, E. J. S. (2020). Institutionalisation and deinstitutionalisation of children 2: Policy and practice recommendations for global, national, and local actors. *Lancet Child and Adolescent Health, 4*, 606–633. doi: 10.1016/S2352-4642(20)30060-2.

Haskins, R. (2017). *A national campaign to improve foster care*. Washington, DC: The Brookings Institution. Retrieved from: https://www.brookings.edu/research/a-national-campaign-to-improve-foster-care/.

Humphreys, K. L., Esteves, K., Zeanah, K., Fox, N. A., Nelson III, C. A., & Drury, S. S. (2016). Accelerated telomere shortening: Tracking the lasting impact of early institutional care at the cellular level. *Psychiatry Research, 246*, 95–100. doi: 10.1016/j.psychres.2016.09.023.

Hyde, J., & Kammerer, N. (2009). Adolescents' perspectives on placement moves and congregate settings: Complex and cumulative instabilities in out-of-home care. *Children and Youth Services Review, 31*, 265–273. doi: 10.1016/j.childyouth.2008.07.019.

James, S. (2011). What works in group care?—A structured review of treatment models for group homes and residential care. *Children and Youth Services Review, 33*, 308–321. doi: 10.1016/j.childyouth.2010.09.014.

James, S., Alemi, Q., & Zepeda, V. (2013). Effectiveness and implementation of evidence-based practices in residential care settings. *Children and Youth Services Review, 35*, 642–656. doi: 10.1016/j.childyouth.2013.01.007.

Johnson, R., Browne, K., & Hamilton-Giachritsis, C. (2006). Young children in institutional care at risk of harm. *Trauma Violence & Abuse*, 7, 34–60. doi: 10.1177/1524838005283696.

Jones, M. B. (1993). Decline of the American orphanage, 1941-1980. *Social Services Review, 67*, 459–480. doi: 10.1086/603999.

Lear, J. (1998). *Open minded: Working out the logic of the soul.* Cambridge, MA: Harvard University Press.

Lee, B. R., & Thompson, R. (2009). Examining externalizing behavior trajectories of youth in group homes: Is there evidence for peer contagion? *Journal of Abnormal Child Psychology*, 37, 31–44. doi: 10.1007/s10802-008-9254-4.

Macarov, D. (2008). Families versus institutions: A global view. *Social Development Issues, 30*, 102–116. Retrieved from: https://web.p.ebscohost.com/ehost/pdfviewer/pdfviewer?vid=0&sid=3781823f-5e36-4141-ab98-d92b9a25f703%40redis.

McCall, J. N. (1999). Research on the psychological effects of orphanage care: A critical review. In R. B. McKenzie (Ed.), *Rethinking orphanages in the 21st century* (pp. 127–150). Thousand Oaks, CA: Sage.

McCrae, J. S., Lee, B. R., Barth, R. P., & Rauktis, M. E. (2010). Comparing three years of well-being outcomes for youth in group care and nonkinship foster care. *Child Welfare*, *89*, 229–249. PMID: 20857889.

McKenzie, R. (1997). Orphanage alumni: How they have done and how they evaluate their experience. *Child & Youth Care Forum*, *26*, 87–111. doi: 10.1007/BF02589359.

McKenzie, R. B. (2003). The impact of orphanages on the alumni's lives and assessments of their childhoods. *Children and Youth Services Review*, *25*, 703–753. doi: 10.1016/S0190-7409(03)00068-9.

Moore, T., McArthur, M., Death, J., Tilbury, C., & Roche, S. (2017). Young people's views on safety and preventing abuse and harm in residential care: "It's got to be better than home." *Children and Youth Services Review*, *81*, 212–219. doi: 10.1016/j.childyouth.2017.08.010.

Moore, T., McArthur, M., Death, J., Tilbury, C., & Roche, S. (2018). Sticking with us through it all: The importance of trustworthy relationships for children and young people in residential care. *Children and Youth Services Review*, *84*, 68–75. doi: 10.1016/j.childyouth.2017.10.043.

Neagu, M. (2021). *Voices from the silent cradles: Life histories of Romania's looked after children*. Bristol: Policy Press.

Nelson, C. A., III, Fox, N. A., & Zeanah, C. H. (2014). *Romania's abandoned children: deprivation, brain development, and the struggle for recovery*. Cambridge, MA: Harvard University Press.

Oliveira, P. S., Fearon, R. M. P., Belsky, J., Fachada, I., & Soares, I. (2015). Quality of institutional care and early childhood development. *International Journal of Behavioral Development*, *39*, 161–170. doi: 10.1177/0165025414552302.

Osei, G. K., & Gorey, K. M. (2019). Peer influences moderated by group home size: Retrospective cohort of youths in Ontario group home care, 2012 to 2016. *Children and Youth Services Review*, *107*, 104564. doi: 10.1016/j.childyouth.2019.104564.

Palmer, L., Ahn, E., Traube, D., Prindle, J., & Putnam-Hornstein, E. (2020). Correlates of entry into congregate care among a cohort of California foster youth. *Children and Youth Services Review*, *110*, 104772. doi: 10.1016/j.childyouth.2020.104772.

Pignotti, M. (2011). Reactive attachment disorder and international adoption: A systematic synthesis. *The Scientific Review of Mental Health Practice*, *8*, 30–49. Retrieved from: https://web.p.ebscohost.com/ehost/pdfviewer/pdfviewer?vid=0&sid=1cc34481-d631-4b86-9a3e-70728f3f71ae%40redis.

Rock, S., Michelson, D., Thomson, S., & Day, C. (2015). Understanding foster placement instability for looked after children: A systematic review and narrative synthesis of quantitative and qualitative evidence. *British Journal of Social Work*, *45*, 177–203. doi: 10.1093/bjsw/bct084.

Ryan, J. P., Marshall, J. M., Herz, D., & Hernandez, P. M. (2008). Juvenile delinquency in child welfare: Investigating group home effects. *Children and Youth Services Review*, *30*, 1088–1099. doi: 10.1016/j.childyouth.2008.02.004.

Sherr, L., Roberts, K. J., & Gandhi, N. (2017). Child violence experiences in institutionalized/orphanage care. *Psychology, Health & Medicine*, *22*, 31–57. doi: 10.1080/13548506.2016.1271951.

Smith, M. (2010). Victim narratives of historical abuse in residential child care do we really know what we think we know? *Qualitative Social Work*, *9*, 303–320. doi: 10.1177/147332501036781.

Stockholm Declaration on Children and Residential Care. (May 2003). Retrieved from: https://resourcecentre.savethechildren.net/pdf/2584.pdf/.

The Leiden Conference on the Development and Care of Children without Permanent Parents. (2012). The development and care of institutionally reared children: Development and care of institutionally reared children. *Child Development Perspectives*, *6*, 174–180. doi: 10.1111/j.1750-8606.2011.00231.x.

The St. Petersburg-USA Orphanage Research Team. (2008). The effects of early social-emotional and relationship experience on the development of young orphanage children. *Monographs of the Society for Research in Child Development*, *73*(3). doi: 10.1002/9781444309683.

Thoburn, J. (2023). Residential care across jurisdictions: Understanding context and comparing data. In J. K. Whittaker, L. Holmes, J. F. del Valle, & S. James (Eds.), *Revitalizing residential care for children and youth: Cross-national trends and challenges* (pp. 16–24). New York: Oxford University Press. doi: 10.1093/oso/9780197644300.003.0002.

van IJzendoorn, M. H., Bakermans-Kranenburg, M., Duchinsky, R., Fox, N. A., Goldman, P. S., Gunnar, M. R., ... Sonuga-Barke, E. J. S. (2020). Institutionalisation and deinstitutionalisation of children 1: A systematic and integrative review of evidence regarding effects on development. *Lancet Psychiatry*, *4*, 1–18. doi: 10.1016/S2215-0366(19)30399-2.

van IJzendoorn, M. H., Luijk, M. P. C. M., & Juffer, F. (2008). Detrimental effects on cognitive development of growing up in children's homes: A meta-analysis on IQ delays in orphanages. *Merrill Palmer Quarterly*, *54*, 341–366. doi: 10.1353/mpq.0.0002.

Wade, M., Parsons, J., Humphreys, K. L., McLaughlin, K. A., Sheridan, K. A., Zeanah, C. H., ... Fox, N. A. (2022). The Bucharest Early Intervention Project: Adolescent mental health and adaptation following early deprivation. *Child Development Perspectives*, *16*, 157–164. doi: 10.1111/cdep.12462.

Wassenaar, D. R. (2006). Commentary: Ethical considerations in international research collaboration: The Bucharest Early Intervention Project. *Infant Mental Health Journal*, 27, 577–580. doi: 10.1002/imhj.20108.

Wastell, D., & White, S. (2012). Blinded by neuroscience: Social policy, the family and the infant brain. *Families, Relationships and Societies*, *1*, 397–414. doi: 10.1332/204674312X656301.

Weiss, B., Caron, A., Ball, S., Tapp, J., Johnson, M., & Weisz, J. R. (2005). Iatrogenic effects of group treatment for antisocial youth. *Journal of Consulting and Clinical Psychology*, *73*, 1036–1044. doi: 10.1037/0022-006X.73.6.1036.

Zeanah, C. H., Fox, N. A., & Nelson, C. A. (2012). Case study in ethics of research: The Bucharest Early Intervention Project. *Journal of Nervous and Mental Disorders*, *200*, 243–247. doi:10.1097/NMD.0b013e318247d275.

5 Explorations of the Effectiveness of Residential Care

The review of literature in Chapter 4 shows that the vigorous campaign to eliminate all residential care for children and youth is not based on research showing that residential care is inherently harmful. Is there reason to believe residential care can be helpful? Perhaps the most important theoretical reason for investing hope in residential care is that quality residential care can provide the two most important things children need: stability and resources (Bornstein, 2015; Ganong, Coleman, & Russell, 2015). The hostility to residential care has led to child welfare systems in the United States and elsewhere that rely on adoption, family reunification, and foster care. Adoption, family reunification, and foster care are to be celebrated when they work, but they do not work in a significant number of cases, sometimes with serious consequences. When foster care does not work, children and youth can be subjected to multiple placements and displacements. Too many foster parents cede custody when children turn out to be difficult to control. The child welfare system has too many children who have had to give up their friends, their schools, and their beds, repeatedly. Placement changes in the double-digits are not uncommon (e.g., Malia, Quigley, Dowty, & Danjczek, 2008; Rock, Michelson, Thomson, & Day, 2015). For those children, good residential care can potentially provide a sense of permanence they have never known. As Holmes, Connolly, Mortimer, and Hevesi (2018) conclude: "...for some young people residential group care can offer the best chance of positive outcomes, transition, and in some cases a route to permanence" (p. 209).

Sources of Support for Residential Care

Have the presuppositions and biases overshadowed evidence that supports residential care? If the conventional wisdom that residential care is inherently harmful is correct, there should be little supportive evidence. Because of the ethical limitations of the research, there is no causal evidence for the efficacy of residential care as there is no causal evidence against residential care. However, there is substantial research to support the use of high-quality residential care (Kendrick, 2013). We will examine five sources that reflect

DOI: 10.4324/9781003435709-5

on the effectiveness of forms of residential care: (a) McKenzie's surveys of alumni of mid-20th century American children's homes; (b) recent international interventions with youth; (c) research directly comparing forms of residential care to alternative forms of care; (d) studies that look at changes during residential care; and (e) a recent review of residential care research from Scotland. Readers are asked to suspend the presumption that residential care is inherently harmful that is based in the infant research and to consider the evidence, some of which has been available for a long time, that residential care can be a positive influence in the lives of children and youth.

Exhibit 1. Richard McKenzie's research with orphanage alumni. In the 1990s, Richard McKenzie brought a unique perspective to the question of the efficacy of residential care. McKenzie, an internationally known economics professor at the University of California at Irvine, spent much of his youth at Barium Springs, a children's home in North Carolina. In a memoir (McKenzie, 1996) McKenzie describes how, from the age of ten, he and his brother lived at the home after his mother died and his alcoholic father could not care for them. McKenzie wrote the memoir after spending his adulthood hearing about how awful orphanages are. He contrasts his experience with what he says the modern foster care system often provides, "...the worst of all forms of care—permanent temporary care" (McKenzie, 1999, p. 1). When he was at Barium Springs, it was a typical early 20th-century American children's home, with a large rural campus where children were taken care of by house parents, ate in a cafeteria, and worked hard on the farm that provided much of the residents' food. Looking back, McKenzie sees the communal nature of Barium Springs and the characteristics it nurtured, especially a strong work ethic and set of morals, as critical in his own development.

McKenzie recognizes that the post-World War II decline in the number of traditional orphanages was due to a complex set of reasons (McKenzie, 1999). Some, including a decline in parent death rates and a decline in poverty, were demographic. Others were reputational, based on Dickensian media depictions and reports of institutional abuse. As a conservative economist, McKenzie also sees the hand of bureaucratic government in the decline as control over children shifted from small, local institutions to government-operated child welfare from a distance. He also blames, without providing evidence, what he calls "self-interested lobbying of social workers" who gained jobs in the monitoring of children in foster care. He does not see his experience as idyllic, but he does wonder "Doesn't anyone (other than the orphanage alumni) understand the value of permanence and stability to children?" (McKenzie, 1999, p. 18).

During the 1990s and early 2000s, McKenzie dedicated some of his prolific research and writing to child welfare. In addition to his memoir, he contributed an edited volume touting the advantages of the heirs of Barium Springs (McKenzie, 1999), an edited volume on the history of orphanages (McKenzie, 2009), and several opinion articles (e.g., McKenzie, 2018). Of particular interest here is his survey research (McKenzie, 1997, 2003). In 1995 McKenzie surveyed orphanage alumni from nine orphanages. He surveyed alumni from five more in 2002. The orphanages were "classic" American orphanages of the mid-20th century. All but one was large (300–400 residents). Children typically were housed in cottages with a single "housemother" and eight to 30 other children. Each home had a farm or large garden where residents worked both during the school year and summers. All the responses he uses in his main reporting come from residents who had left the orphanage setting by 1967, when many of the institutions had closed or morphed into different kinds of service organizations. Using the same eight-page, 56 question survey in both studies, he obtained over 2,000 usable responses from the two surveys with a nearly 50% response rate, unusually high for such uncompensated and comprehensive surveys. McKenzie's reports are long, so I will summarize the general findings and leave the details to the curious.

The findings from the two surveys are strikingly similar so I will note differences only when they are major. The alumni had entered the orphanage sometime between infancy and age 17 years, with a mean of about eight years. Most left the orphanage at 17 or 18 having spent about eight years there on average. They responded to the survey in their 40s to their 80s. Relatively few had lost both parents. They were all white. Respondents were above average (compared to census data for whites of the same age) in high school and college graduation rates and those in the first survey were more likely to hold an advanced degree. Respondents from the first survey and those above age 55 in the second survey had above average incomes. Few respondents had ever been incarcerated and fewer than 6% reported ever being on public assistance. In response to the question "All things considered, how would you say things are going for you these days?" McKenzie's respondents were much more likely than average to indicate that they were "very happy." The only question on which respondents indicated more trouble than average was concerning divorce rates. In both sets of survey responses there was a higher likelihood of divorce among the former residents.

Across surveys, when asked whether they would have preferred foster care to living in the orphanage, they overwhelmingly said they would have chosen the orphanage over a foster care placement. Few reported thinking about being adopted. About half wanted to go back to their family of origin "sometimes" or "frequently," but a quarter said they never did. On open-ended questions, the negatives about the orphanages listed most commonly were separation from family members, a lack of emotional support, and a lack of freedom. A quarter of the respondents indicated that there were "no problems." Positives from the residential experience listed by respondents included acquiring personal values and direction, education and guidance, spiritual values, and a sense of self-worth.

McKenzie appropriately points out the weaknesses of the survey method. Those who responded may have been those who had the most positive experiences and positive outcomes, a problem in follow-ups of alumni of any organization. Respondents tend to have selective memory for more positive experience (Prebble, Addis, & Tippett, 2013). Generalization (external validity) of his findings is problematic because of populations and settings differences and changes over time. The positive findings in this case, however, were found for children and youth who had been in environments that were, on average, less advantageous than those children and youth in residential care typically experience now. McKenzie may be being kind when he concludes that the common descriptions of orphanage environments as irredeemably depriving "...have been far too sweeping, all-inclusive, or without adequate recognition of the variation in the quality of care provided" (McKenzie, 2003, p. 738).

McKenzie starts both reports on his 1995 survey with a quote (already quoted in Chapter 4 regarding hostility) from two authors who were writing for the North American Council on Adoptable Children: "fifty years of research reconfirms the same findings: long-term institutionalization in childhood leads to recurrent problems in interpersonal relationships, a high rate of personality disorders, and severe parenting difficulties late in life" (McKenzie, 1999, p. 87). We saw in Chapters 2 and 4 that the "50 years of research showing residential care is detrimental" is ephemeral. McKenzie's survey results suggest that such broad statements are indefensible. We are not talking here about late 20th-century or early 21st-century children's homes with small, stable adult-child ratios, special education opportunities, and limited chore schedules. McKenzie's data on educational attainments, general reports of happiness, and memories of their residential upbringings show that even institutions that would be seen as inappropriate today did not do psychological harm and, instead, apparently provided environments for young people to develop normally or even advantageously.

Survey research, with its measurement and sampling limitations, may not be impressive. There are no sophisticated psychological measures or experimental designs. McKenzie just asked former residents about their experiences. Simple and powerful. Not all former residents of Barium Springs were as positive as McKenzie about their experience. Campbell (2000), a true orphan and a 1956 graduate of Barium Springs High School who had spent 15 of his first 17 years at the home and subsequently became a college professor too reported a more mixed experience. Yet he concluded his memoir with this:

> Almost to a person, I was surrounded by caring individuals who provided for me and sheltered me from the temptations, pushes, and pulls of society. And I have come to believe that the next best substitute for my biological family was Barium Springs Home For Children. And I will be forever grateful for my home.
>
> (p. 102)

We do need to be cautious about generalizing McKenzie's findings to today's residential care. Residents in his research were often in care for different reasons; few were there after multiple foster family placements. Yet his evidence is a better fit than that provided by those who make sweeping overgeneralizations about every kind of residential care from research on infants in Romanian orphanages. More important, McKenzie's data are more pertinent to the remaining forms of residential care in many countries than data from on infants from severely deprived environments. As McKenzie readily admits, among the classic orphanages there undoubtedly were institutions that should have been closed before they were. Their modern counterparts are probably better places for children and youth. But based on self-reports, they did not damage the majority of their residents and apparently enhanced the physical, social-psychological, and educational development of most. There are many reasons why the classic orphanages disappeared in the United States, not least because of expense and often due to undeserved bad reputations. It was not because of accumulated research evidence that they harmed their charges.

Why have McKenzie's arguments gotten so little traction in child welfare scholardom? Even when cited, they are sometimes misrepresented as McKenzie indicated in footnote 9 (p. 709) of his 2003 paper. One problem is timing. McKenzie conducted his first survey during a national debate about welfare that included an argument by prominent right-wing conservative Newt Gingrich of "Contract with America" fame for using orphanages to raise the children of unwed welfare mothers. The Dickensian orphanage theme was revived as child advocates recoiled in horror. McKenzie's association with right wing economic and political thought probably did not help. Another factor working against McKenzie was his description of the Barium Springs orphanage in his memoir. It emphasized old-fashioned, conservative values like hard work and moral development. The number of hours per week children and youth worked would be seen by many in the 1990s as abusive. By the mid-1990s, the demonization of residential care had become an unstated presupposition of many in the child welfare field. For instance, in response to the Gingrich kerfuffle, the New York official largely responsible for closing the state's orphanages in the 1960s and 1970s, Barbara Bloom, was quoted in the Los Angeles Times as saying "They [orphanages] were not appropriate places for children to develop mentally. The *evidence was so blatant* that we assumed we'd never revisit the issues" (Shogren & Mehren, 1994, December 26, A1, my emphasis). Finally, the welfare debates of the 1990s were accompanied by an almost religious belief in the sanctity of the biological family. McKenzie was fighting that ingrained ideology along with what Gelles (1999) called "...a nearly missionary marketing of the virtues of intensive family preservation services" (p. 49). That zeal for the efficacy of fixing families has not yet been dampened by the evidence from randomized clinical trials that demonstrate that families are hard to change (e.g., Bezeczky et al., 2020; Schweitzer, Pecora, Nelson, Walters, & Blythe, 2015; but see Huhr & Wulczyn, 2022 for signs of hope, at least with families with very young children). It is a central tenet of the Family First Prevention Services Act of 2018.

The last paragraph of McKenzie's (1996) memoir is apt:

> Today's disadvantaged children need a break. They need love and nurturing. When those precious advantages cannot be provided, children need, at a minimum, a safe, stable, structured, and permanent place that provides opportunities for personal growth, a chance to live down and away from the problems of their past. They need the break I was lucky enough to get at the Home.
>
> (p. 228)

McKenzie may have been a little naïve about how his particular vision of residential care, based on his own experience, could be reproduced in the 21st century. But he has visited some of the heirs of homes like Barium Springs and has seen how improvements in quality have made it possible to work with young people who are much more challenging than he and his peers were. McKenzie's contribution to the child welfare literature is to call the bluff of those who claim: "all the research evidence shows how horrible every residential environment is for children and youth of all ages" or that "children not brought up in a family are doomed."

Exhibit 2. Duke's Positive Outcomes for Orphans studies and OSCAR. The question of care for children and youth in need of parents is particularly complex when considered globally. UNICEF estimates that over two million children live in "institutions" worldwide (https://data.unicef.org/topic/child-protection/children-alternative-care/). If the conventional negative view of residential care so widely held in child welfare is accurate, are these children relegated to lives of suboptimal development? Do the negative outcomes from studies of infants developing in the extremely deprived environments in Romania and similar institutions apply to these older children and youth in a wide variety of group settings? Are children whose parents cannot take care of them always better off in a family setting than in a residential environment?

The Duke Global Health Institute has an interest in many aspects of health and wellbeing of children around the world. Their Positive Outcomes for Orphans (POFO) study (Whetten et al., 2009) directly addresses the issues of concern to us. Its cohort includes a large group of single- and double-orphans from six culturally diverse sites in five low- and middle-income countries: Cambodia, Ethiopia, Kenya, India, and Tanzania. The orphans, ages six to 12 years at the start of the study, were from either one of 83 institutions or families (1,357) from one of 311 community clusters in the same area as most were in some form of kinship care. The "institutions" ranged from very large ones (376 children) to smaller ones that were more like group homes (with five to ten children). Measures of physical growth (height, weight, BMI), general health (caregiver ratings), emotional health (the Strengths and Difficulties Questionnaires), and learning ability and memory (Kaufman Assessment Battery for Children-II subtests) were obtained. The study's original hypothesis, based on the conventional wisdom was that all institutions negatively affect the development of those who reside in them and that the children in families would fare better across measures. The results of the study show that, contrary to conventional wisdom, children in kinship care did not fare better than those in institutional care. There was much more variability within the groups than between the groups.

In a follow-up with the cohort three years later (Whetten et al., 2014), the same set of measures was administered. Of the original group of 2,837 children, 2,283 completed the three-year follow-up assessment (data from the original assessment are reported in detail in Whetten et al., 2009); 1,290 children from families and 993 residing in institutions. Only three group differences were found. Children in institutions were taller and healthier (according to caregiver reports of physical conditions) than those in families and had fewer caregiver-reported emotional difficulties. As in the original study, within group variability (differences between children within families and institutions) was much greater than differences between children in the two groups. The variable of "where children lived" during the three years between assessments did not account for individual changes in any meaningful way. Perhaps what is most clear from this study is that the hypothesis that living in a residential institution would adversely affect children's wellbeing was not supported. The authors conclude that the way to increase outcomes for the greatest number of children is to improve the quality of the children's experiences in both family and residential care settings.

Further analysis of the third-year follow-up is reported by Huynh et al. (2019). They looked at child wellbeing as measured by the Strengths and Difficulties Questionnaire as a function of four factors from the Child Status Index: food insecurity, shelter adequacy, health care, and caregiving quality (adult physical and psychological security and support). They report that all four child status factors were related to child wellbeing, but that the factors did not interact with site of care (family or residential setting). They conclude:

> Child psychosocial well-being across "high" and "low" levels of quality of care showed negligible differences between residential- and community-based care settings, suggesting the important factor in child well-being is quality of care rather than setting of care.
>
> (Huynh et al., 2019, p. 1)

In other research with the cohort, Gray et al. (2015) describe self-reported potentially traumatic event results from the Life Events Checklist for those in institutions and families. Children from both settings reported high incidences of potentially traumatic events and there was no setting difference overall. However, reported incidents of physical or sexual abuse were more common by children in family settings. At a follow-up at 90 months (Gray et al., 2016), those members of the cohort 16 years or older reported on their sexual health. Fewer than 10% of the adolescents reported having engaged in sex by age 15. However, among those who did, recent intercourse (within the past year) and unprotected sex were more common among those who were living in families.

The Duke studies are important. The studies suffer from the typical problem of under-describing the nature of the children's experiences. It is unlikely that most of the institutions come close to being the kind of high-quality residential care described in Chapters 6 and 7 of this book. There is no complete control for systematic differences in the groups. However, the studies involved a large number of children, the comparison groups were carefully selected, they used a wide array of physical and psychological measures of demonstrable reliability and validity, and, perhaps most important, the research program includes a longitudinal component with a high retention rate. The results directly contradict the implications of the classic studies of infants in extremely deprived environments and the conventional wisdom about residential care inferred from those studies. Even in institutional environments that are very different than those found in advantaged countries today, children can thrive, even relative to their family-based peers.

In a study similar to the Duke work, Embleton et al. (2014) outline different forms of care for orphaned and separated children in Kenya as part of the OSCAR (Orphaned & Separated Children's Assessments Related to their Health & Well-Being Project) study (https://oscarcohort.com/the-oscar-study/), a cooperative venture of investigators from Moi University in Kenya, Indiana University in the United States, and other institutions. In a detailed analysis of the independent variable (the type of care) that is so rare in this literature, they carefully describe the alternative settings and how each setting affords opportunities within a children's human rights framework (the ten articles of the United Nations Convention on the Rights of the Child). They do so in response to the call of UNICEF, Save the Children, and others to de institutionalize the care of all children of all ages. Those calls identify institutional care as child abuse. They do so without a base in empirical research to indicate all institutional care is abusive. The OSCAR study focuses on Charitable Children's Institutions (CCIs), community organizations (essentially day cares), and households where children were taken care of by a surviving parent, extended family members, or others (formal or informal foster care). Their basic finding is that the care in the institutions is more likely to meet the basic rights requirements of the United Nations Convention than the family care studied. Overall, those in charitable institutions were doing better than children living with extended family in the community. Children in charitable institutions were more likely to have their basic nutritional needs met, were more likely to have books and other educational resources, were more likely to have advanced medical care, were less likely to be subjected to corporal punishment, and were less likely to be subject to intrusive amounts of labor. The study points to concrete ways that care in households can be supplemented and improved, but many extended families, especially those dealing with HIV in their families, are simply overwhelmed and have difficulty providing basic resources.

The lesson of the Duke and OSCAR research is that there are advantages and disadvantages of different modes of care. In a complex world where children live in very different environments, a wide range of options is needed. Eliminating any one mode without evidence to support its elimination is not warranted. Since before the 1909 White House Conference on Children those in the United States who considered themselves "progressive" or "reformist" have seen residential care as a last resort, particularly for infants. Residential care was often a last resort for children who lived in poverty (when 50% of working-class families were poor), not children who were true orphans or came from seriously troubled families. The number of children in residential care declined dramatically when other means of helping the poor were developed, such as the federal Aid for Dependent Children in the United States (Jones, 1993). Perhaps something similar eventually will occur in the countries studied by those at Duke and OSCAR.

Exhibit 3. A review of "direct" comparisons between group care and alternatives. Studies of developmental outcomes from group care versus alternatives are rare. The ones that exist often suffer from serious methodological deficiencies. The most serious problems concern small sample sizes, non-equivalent groups, and a failure to sufficiently describe the nature of the group care (and/or, in some cases, the alternative care). Sometimes the group care is not actually residential care, but some form of short-term shelter care. An important review by Lee, Bright, Svoboda, Fakunmoju, and Barth (2011) includes 19 different studies. Three compare some form of group care to family foster care. Eight compare group care to therapeutic foster care, three group care to non-placement, and five compare an older model of group care to a newer one. The eight studies of group care versus therapeutic foster care represent only two different research groups. In several cases, separate publications use the same sample, reporting on results from different measures or measures taken at different times. All told, fewer than ten of the studies represent independent findings of some form of group care versus an alternative.

One of the three studies comparing **group care and foster care**, DeSena et al. (2005), used an intervention (called SAFE Homes) designed to reduce "foster care drift" (the tendency for children and youth to drift from one placement to another without any clear plan for permanency). Individuals were kept in a shelter for 45 days before first placement to undergo detailed assessments with the aim of developing assessment-based permanency plans. Both groups had 342 children aged three to 12 years, matched using propensity scores (a technique that statistically pairs children from two groups on a variety of demographic and other variables). The 11 outcome measures include how long participants were in out-of-home care, whether they were placed with siblings and when, costs, and number of placements at various intervals. Five of the 11 comparisons show statistically significant differences, all but one (initial placement with siblings) favoring family foster care. The stated focus of the study was the efficacy of the SAFE intervention. Essentially, it did not work. The state (California) had already made major improvements in its placement procedures independent of the study, making it unlikely the intervention would do better.

The second study comparing group care and foster care reviewed by Lee et al. is Friedrich, Baker, Parker, Schneiderman, Gries, and Archer's (2005) examination of the stability of problematic sexual behavior among ten- to 12-year-olds over a year in residential treatment center (39 children) or in family foster care (43 children). Problematic sexual behavior persisted more for those in the residential treatment program. The strength of the result is attenuated by the fact that the most disturbed children had been placed in the treatment center. Regardless of group placement, those with initial problematic sexual behavior were likely to have similar levels a year later. The third, archival, study comparing group care with foster care (Ryan et al., 2008) reports results with a very large group of youth in Los Angeles County. The focal research question is whether youth who spent time in residential care were more likely than those who had not to have later trouble with law enforcement (i.e., been arrested). All the children and youth were between seven and 16 years of age. The type of care is not detailed but fell in "a broad category of residential care," including "half-way homes, campus-based homes, emergency shelters, self-contained settings, and staff secured setting (sic)" (p. 1088). The researchers found a small effect size favoring those who had not ever been in group care. Their two explanations for the difference are group contagion or a lower threshold for reporting misbehavior leading to arrest by staff at group homes compared to foster families. Two problems with the study are that most placements in group homes resulted from foster parents being unwilling to continue with the placement and the utter lack of any kind of description of the residential care or differences in the quality of care.

Of the eight publications Lee et al. report on that compare **group care with therapeutic foster care**, seven were conducted at the Oregon Social Learning Center with adolescent boys or girls (Chamberlain & Reid, 1998; Chamberlain, Leve, & DeGarmo, 2007; Eddy & Chamberlain, 2000; Eddy, Whaley, & Chamberlain, 2004; Kerr, Leve, & Chamberlain, 2009; Leve & Chamberlain, 2007; Leve, Chamberlain, & Reid, 2005). The youth, 12–19 years of age, had histories of serious and chronic delinquency. In each of the papers, a study is reported on how youth did in a family foster care home where parents had been trained in intense multidimensional treatment foster care methods and were closely supervised compared to how youth did in one of many group homes (ranging from 11 to 35 different group homes per publication). The therapeutic care parents were trained in providing clear limit setting, mentoring behaviors, controlling access to delinquent peers, recognizing anxiety, and strategies for increasing emotional regulation and decreasing social aggression. The only description of what went on in the many group homes was that most used some version of Positive Peer Culture.

Different dependent variables were used in the seven Oregon reports (some of the papers reported on follow-ups of previous studies). They included program completion, runaways, days in lockups, arrests, criminal referrals, self-reports of delinquent behavior, and school achievement. In one of the studies of adolescent girls, pregnancies were counted. Across the Oregon studies, youth in multidimensional treatment foster care did better than those in group homes. On 28 measures, the multidimensional treatment foster care group did significantly better. The statistical effect sizes ranged from 0.36 to 0.79 (small to moderate).

The only non-Oregon study comparing group care with therapeutic foster care is from Girls and Boys Town (Lee & Thompson, 2008). It provides very different results than those from the Oregon studies. Children and youth eight years and above in family-style residential care (numbering 112) were matched using propensity scores to children and youth in treatment foster care. Based on two-tailed statistical tests (tests that do not presuppose the direction of a difference favoring either group), the results show those in treatment foster care were less likely than those in residential care to be favorably discharged, less likely to return home, and more likely to experience formal institutional placements later. There were no differences on legal involvement or likelihood of residing in a homelike setting six months after discharge.

Three studies reviewed by Lee et al. compared children in **group care with those who received non-placement services.** Barth, Greeson, Guo, Green, Duppong Hurley, and Sisson (2007) compared residential care (a "good program") with in-home therapy. There was no significant difference between groups on a composite outcome measure of family stability, legal issues, education, and out-of-home placements after discharge. The other two studies in this category favored residential care. Byrnes, Hansen, Malloy, Carter, and Curry (1999) conducted two studies comparing results from day treatment and residential care for juvenile offenders. In the first study, there were no differences in quarterly rates of offending (although both groups showed reductions in criminal charges). In the second study of another group, those who had been in residential care were less likely than those who had received day treatment to evidence adult convictions. The Thompson et al. (1996) report is another study from Boys Town (now Girls and Boys Town). Focusing on educational outcomes, they compared youth who resided at Boys Town with a group that had been admitted to Boys Town but did not attend for various reasons. On all four educationally related measures (GPA, school records, positive attitudes, and years completed), those who had resided at Boys Town did better. In a similar, more recent study in Denmark, youth who completed secondary school while in residential care were more likely than those in foster care to employed or in an education or training at age 25 (Lausten, 2023).

The five studies in the last group Lee et al. include in their review do not speak directly to the question of the effects of residential care, instead comparing **different forms of group care.** The two studies in this set that included pre- and post-measures show improvement in both forms of care studied (Deschenes & Greenwood, 1998; Mann-Feder, 1996).

Except for the Oregon studies, differences between types of care in the studies reviewed by Lee et al. are small. The participants in the studies represent a very heterogenous group, although a majority of the study participants were juvenile offenders. The failure to specify the nature of the group care in most of these studies is particularly troublesome. The programs studied ranged from wilderness programs to traditional lockdown custodial units. Issues of quality of care simply are not addressed. Given these limitations, some highly tentative conclusions are that: (a) family foster care works slightly better than community group homes; (b) therapeutic foster care works better than community group homes with juvenile offenders; and (c) high-quality children's homes (Boy's Town and Barth et al.'s "good program") are as effective or more effective than therapeutic foster care or non-placement services.

An alternative, more recent review of residential care versus therapeutic foster care is reported by Gutterswijk et al. (2020). However, there are significant problems with this work. The investigators conducted a meta-analysis of 24 studies that compared the Treatment Foster Care Oregon for Adolescents or one of four types of home-based treatment to "residential care." It is the ubiquitous problem of the meaning of residential care in this analysis that is particularly problematic. The authors note the limitation of not knowing important characteristics of the residential care such as level of security, available treatments within the care, or even size of the residential unit. However, the meaning of residential care in this report is problematical at the macro level. The 24 studies include high-security correctional facilities, psychiatric hospitals, short-term (two weeks or less) emergency care, and group homes. Gutterswijk and his colleagues expected the analysis would favor non-residential care because residential care does not allow for self-determination, provides involvement with deviant peers, risks institutional repression, does not provide evidence-based treatment, separates residents from attachment relationships, and there are problems in establishing youth-staff relationships. Of course, all of those vary considerably in different kinds of residential care and also in family care.

The investigators report 145 effect sizes. Effect sizes are statistical indicators of how much the average (mean) score of a group differs from the average (mean) in another group, accounting for how much variability there is within the groups. A mean difference between any two groups is relatively less important if there is a lot of variability in the scores. Gutterswijk et al. (2020) report about six effect sizes per "study" (i.e., publication). However, three papers provide 53 of the 145 effect sizes and six others provide 23, together accounting for half of the effect sizes. The researchers argue that their three-level meta-analysis (checking on sample variance, within study variance, and between study variance) allows control for statistical dependencies. However, when combined with heterogeneous dependent and independent variables, those conceptual dependencies make the modest finding of the study difficult to interpret. That modest finding is a slightly more positive outcome in the home-based care. Note that Gutterwijk et al. do not find that residential care, even of this extremely mixed sort, including highly restrictive care, is inherently harmful.

Exhibit 4. Pre-post change: Do children and youth get worse in residential care? Studies simply assessing children and youth when they enter residential care and later are common in the residential care literature. Causal conclusions about the effectiveness of care cannot be made by looking at pre-post change. However, if residential care is as uniformly harmful as the conventional wisdom suggests, children and youth experiencing residential care should show consistent deterioration in their wellbeing while in care and should not show improvements. Many of the studies of pre-post change among older children and adults have been conducted with youth offenders or those with serious emotional or behavioral problems. Studies of pre-post change in children's homes or group homes are rare. We will look in detail at two review projects (Knorth, Harder, Zandberg, & Kendrick, 2008; James, 2011) and two studies (Nixon & Henderson, 2022; Portwood, Boyd, & Murdock, 2016) that represent the available pre-post literature well (Portwood et al., 2018 reports on a subset of those included in the 2016 study and obtained similar results).

Knorth et al. (2008) starts with an indication of the authors' surprise at the difference pointed out by Anglin and Knorth (2004) between declarations from conferences about residential care held in Sweden less than 15 years apart. The earlier Malmö Conference statement concluded that residential care had developed into "a really qualified and efficient aid to education in recent years," and should be considered a "comparable provision for those whom it was appropriate and desirable, not as a last resort" (Anglin & Knorth, 2004, p. 124). Referring to the later Stockholm declaration, Knorth et al. (2008) asked: Is it 'indisputable' that youth mainly experience negative consequences of a residential stay and get worse? (p. 124).

To answer that question, Knorth et al. conducted a meta-analysis of studies published between 1990 and 2005 in the child welfare and related literature. Their original set of 138 identified studies was reduced to 27 by incrementally applying criteria necessary for use in meta-analyses. Of the 138, 14 did not focus on the impact of residential care, 14 repeated results that would have led to double-counting non-independent statistics, 46 did not have pre- and post-data, and 37 did not use the same samples or instruments pre- and post-treatment, did not use reliable, valid instruments, or did not provide the statistical information needed to be used in a meta-analysis. All of these limitations demonstrate the sad state of this research literature. The authors note:

> ...in a large majority (83%) of the 110 studies we analyzed, the residential care program that is subject of research is merely described in global terms, or not described at all. In much of the research the intervention

> package remains too much of a 'black box' (Axford et al., 2005). On this point there is still a lot of work to do.
>
> (Knorth et al., 2008, p. 137)

It is the ten pre-experimental designs that are of interest here (Knorth et al.'s Table 5, pp. 130–131). They provide data on pre-post change over time. The other quasi-experimental studies almost all made comparisons of groups receiving different types of care and did not provide evidence on within group change.

The ten included pre-experimental design studies were on 840 youth 12–18 years of age, most of whom were in either residential care for offenders (custodial care) or psychiatric care (therapeutic residential care). Measures were generally of short-term effects, not longitudinal patterns. Five of the studies report results on problem behavior (some version or versions of the Child Behavior Checklist), including externalizing (acting out) and internalizing (emotionally withdrawn) behaviors. Two of those studies also report results from measures of general psychosocial functioning. Two other studies report results just for psychosocial functioning (but not problem behavior) and one reports on reading skills.

For problem behaviors, the weighted effect size (positive effect sizes indicate improvement over time) was +0.60 (five studies), for externalizing, +0.60 (five studies), and for internalizing, +0.45 (seven studies). The individual study effect sizes ranged from –0.15 to +1.29. Of the 24 individual effect sizes, 18 were positive. There were not enough common measures to generate overall effect sizes for psychosocial functioning. For individual measures, effect sizes ranged from –0.93 to +2.00. Of the 15 effect sizes, 14 were positive. The one negative effect size was for adolescents with conduct disorder diagnoses on a measure of reciprocal family interactions (i.e., they got worse based on a brief set of survey items). Both measures of reading in the remaining study showed slight improvement.

Although the studies in the Knorth et al. review have many limitations, the investigators' conclusion is clear:

> The main conclusion that can be made from our meta-analysis is that children and youth, after a period of residential care – on average – improve in their psychosocial functioning. The "indisputable evidence" that this form of care has (mainly) negative consequences for individual children and for the society at large, as stated in the Stockholm Declaration, has not been supported.
>
> (Knorth et al., 2008, p. 133)

In an overview of treatment models for residential care, James (2011) summarizes the state of the literature at that time: "The outcome literature on group care is scant, and current knowledge about its effect on targeted outcomes is mostly based on studies with small nonrepresentative samples, and weak study designs, lacking control groups and standardized measures" (p. 308). With that caveat, James attempts to disambiguate the independent (treatment) variable by looking closely at the treatment model used in those programs that have been studied with at least a pre-post design. She found evidence on five treatment models in the peer-reviewed literature at that time. Using the California Evidence-based Clearinghouse for Child Welfare criteria for effectiveness, she evaluates the five programs for their relevance to child welfare populations and outcomes and for the scientific evidence supporting their effectiveness. It is the latter ratings that are of most concern here. To receive the highest rating ("well-supported by research evidence"), a program would have to: (a) show no potential risk for harm; (b) have procedures and practices specified in a way that would be exportable, such as in a book or manual; (c) have been positively evaluated in at least two randomized clinical trials at two different sites with results published in peer-reviewed journals; (d) have support from at least one peer-reviewed study that showed results lasting at least one year; (e) have been evaluated using reliable and valid outcome measures; and (f) the overall weight of evidence from peer-reviewed studies supports the effectiveness of the intervention. Lower ratings were attached to programs with less well-specified practices and procedures, fewer supporting randomized clinical trials or research using pre-experimental designs, and/or less reliable and valid measures.

I will have more to say about the details of two models of residential care in Chapter 7. Here the issue is evidence of pre-post change that indicates harm or benefit from residential care. I will follow the order in which James examines the five models. Note that most of the research reviewed here does not compare some form of residential care to non-residential care. Our concern is whether there is evidence for positive or negative change in indicators in well-being during the time children and youth are in care.

The **Positive Peer Culture** treatment method focuses on turning negative peer cultures into ones that foster prosocial behavior, self-esteem, censure of maladaptive behaviors, and the development of community. James identified three peer reviewed articles on Positive Peer Culture in residential care, one experimental and two quasi-experimental. All three were studies done in youth correctional facilities (custodial care). None of the studies included non-residential care control groups. The studies, including the one with the experimental design, reported only differences in change between a treatment group and a control group. Almost all reported change scores on social skills, self-reported anti-social behavior, and self-concept were positive, even for the control groups.

James reviews two studies of the **Teaching Family Model** in residential settings with youth offenders. One showed significant improvement in two measures of behavior problems with youth performing near national norms at a three-month follow-up. The other study showed significant reductions in the use of physical restraints and negative incident reports over a two-year period. In three other quasi-experimental studies of the Teaching Family Model, youth offenders showed improvements on measures of overall adjustment and relationships with others and decreases in offenses after discharge. They also showed improvements on a variety of educational measures. While those in homes using the Teaching Family Model showed more positive change, even those in other homes showed improvement. Of particular note is the Thompson et al. (1996) study (reviewed in Exhibit 3, above) of nearly 500 alumni of Boys Town (which uses the Teaching Family Model) compared to 84 youth who were admitted to Boys Town but who did not attend. In an eight-year follow-up, the Boys Town alumni had higher grades, completed more years of school, and were more likely to attend college. Thompson et al. conclude: "It is suggested that long-term educational effects with troubled children may require an intensive intervention over an extended period of time" (p. 221).

The **Sanctuary Model** was originally developed by Sandra Bloom as a short-term treatment for psychiatric patients. It is a trauma-informed approach for changing organizational cultures to make them more developmental, nonviolent, open, and democratic. On a variety of standardized measures, including the Child Behavior Checklist, measures of self-esteem, locus of control, social problem solving, and coping, that "differences in improvement" ($p < 0.05$) were found in comparison to non-Sanctuary programs six months after intake.

Designed for children and youth in residential treatment centers who are in a downward spiral of emotional and behavioral disorder, the **Stop-Gap Model** provides intense interventions for as short a period as possible. The intent is to return individuals to their communities (the least restrictive environment) quickly. Residents are provided with environments, from token economies to anger management, with increasingly fewer barriers and that target skills that help reduce problem behaviors. At the time of James' review, only data from the original study were available. In a quasi-experimental study, compared to 25 adolescent women in traditional residential treatment, 25 women in the Stop-Gap condition had a lower mean number of "therapeutic holds," but pre-post data were not provided.

Re-ED is an acronym for Re-education of Children with Emotional Disturbance a model with roots in the work of Nicholas Hobbs (1966). The model emphasizes the strengths of children and youth, focusing on the development of skills, competencies, and relationships. It is designed for work with eight to ten individuals for short times several times a day. Individuals remain in residence for four to six months and then return to their communities.

James found only three peer-reviewed studies, all of which employed pre-post designs without comparison groups. The oldest study (Weinstein, 1969) provides pre-post data on 250 children with an average age of eight years when first seen. Specially trained teachers, not psychiatrists, psychologists, or social workers worked with the children. When referring agency personnel or the children's parents rated the improvement of the children, 73%–89% rated the children "moderately" or "greatly" improved. Children showed significant improvement on 15 of 20 measures of psychological wellbeing. At a six-month follow-up after discharge, teachers in their communities rated them significantly improved in behavior and achievement. Similar results were found in a later study of Re-ED with children ages six to 12 years in a state-run residential treatment program who had been diagnosed with ADHD, externalizing behavior problems, or mood disorders (Fields, Farmer, Apperson, Mustillo, & Simmers., 2006). Children showed improvement on measures of problem behaviors and social skills at discharge and at a follow-up. Younger children improved the most and longer stays were correlated with more positive outcomes.

Based on James' review of studies of what happens to children and youth while in residential care, it is difficult to attribute harm to residential care. Positive outcomes are the norm. Like in the Knorth et al. (2008) review, the "indisputable evidence" view that residential care has negative consequences for children is not supported.

Most of the data in the James review came from residential treatment programs for youthful offenders. The advantage of the Portwood et al. (2016) study is that it includes a much broader range of forms of residential care. Their work may provide the best evidence yet against the myth of inevitable detrimental effects of residential care. In their introduction, the investigators review a set of studies comparing residential care to other options that they deemed to be inconclusive for a number of reasons. Residential care is seen as less favorable only because it is more expensive (Lee et al., 2011). Portwood et al.'s purpose is to examine the effectiveness of residential services across a wide variety of programs serving public systems (mental health, child welfare, court) and private (family) referrals. Their sample of programs comes from 37 different agencies in two states. The research process itself was incorporated into the agencies' practice rather than being imposed by the investigators. Portwood et al. hypothesized that children and youth who were already high functioning (i.e., they entered care with non-clinical levels of functioning) would maintain those levels while those with low levels of functioning at intake would show improvements.

The children and youth studied included 184 eight- to ten-year-olds and 930 11- to 17-year-olds. Most were Caucasian (58.4%) or African American (31.9%). The state department of social services had legal custody of 55.4% and parents 37.2%. A major advantage of this study is that it uses a variety of reliable and valid measures of child and youth functioning. They include the Children's Global Assessment Scale (CGAS), an indicator of overall psychological health completed by clinicians (usually therapists or caseworkers), the Achenbach Child Behavior Checklist, a measure of internalizing and externalizing problem behaviors, completed by trained staff members, and a form of the Achenbach completed by the youth themselves (those 11 years or older). Data were obtained at intake, three months after intake, and then at six-month intervals for those who remained in care. Children were separated into high-functioning, low-functioning, or borderline groups based on CGAS intake scores. Approximately a third were in low management residential group care, a quarter in residential treatment, and 14% in high-management residential care.

The results of the study must be qualified due to experimental mortality (two-thirds of the participants were discharged from their particular form of care during the study), missing data, and regression to the mean (the statistical tendency for extreme scores to move toward the middle, the bane of pre-post designs). However, results on the CGAS are clear: "Overall, this series of analyses supported the two study hypotheses, with those demonstrating low levels of global functioning at intake improving across time, and those with non-clinical scores at intake maintaining normal levels of functioning" (p. 402). On the Achenbach (Child Behavior Checklist) completed by professional staff members, internalizing problems decreased for all three groups. Staff-rated externalizing scores increased a small amount for the high-functioning and borderline groups. On the self-reports, there were no changes for internalizing problems and an increase in externalizing problems only for the borderline group. "Taken as a whole, these findings provide empirical support for a number of promising outcomes for children in care; stated differently, there was little evidence that residential care was ineffective" (p. 405). The highest functioning residents showed the least improvement, but they were already scoring in normal ranges of the instruments at intake. Contrary to the myth of inevitable harm, participants did not do worse in residential care and improved on many indicators.

Residential care is used in Scotland for a minority of the children in care. Nixon and Henderson (2022) focus on the youngest group in residential care (those five to 12 years of age). They report on data gathered on 135 children in that age group who were in residential care for extended periods. The children had extensive histories of abuse and neglect and often had been in multiple foster placements before entering residential care. Placement changes were usually due to difficult child behaviors and the inability of foster parents to deal with those behaviors. Administrative referrals and reports from social work, police, school, health professionals, and others were coded on a wide variety of indicators of wellbeing. Records from 12 months before residential care entry, 12 months into care, and 24 months into care were used.

Across a wide variety of coded variables, children in residential care showed consistent improvement. There were declines over time in the proportion of children described as exhibiting self-harm behaviors, suicidal ideation, anger management issues, low self-esteem, sadness, anxiety, conduct disorders, sleep disturbances, and inappropriate sexual behaviors. Children clearly improved while in residential care. The researchers argue that residential care provided children with stability that had not previously characterized their environments.

Overall, the available pre-post data show that children and youth do well in residential care. Results from pre-experimental and quasi-experimental studies cannot "prove" anything. However, strong statements about the inevitable decline of those experiencing residential care are unsupportable when there is no evidence of decline during residence. When children and youth consistently do better rather than worse when they are in residential care, those who say that residential care is inevitably harmful simply cannot be correct.

Exhibit 5: Recent research: The Centre for Excellence for Children's Care and Protection Review. A recent article (Giraldi et al., 2022) and the longer report it is based on (Porter, Giraldi, & Mitchell, 2020) are a review conducted by a Scottish research center and commissioned by an international organization that provides residential care, the SOS Children's Villages. As is so common in this literature, the investigators appear to have started from the stance of the conventional wisdom and are surprised by their results. This may be most obvious from the tortured conclusion the authors reach:

> We found insufficient evidence to substantiate claims that residential care is inherently unsuitable, universally offering low-quality care and negatively impacting children's well-being and developmental outcomes.
> (Giraldi et al., 2022, p. 833)

I have included a summary of their research here because it could have contradicted the other findings reported in the other exhibits and it focuses on recent research reports.

The Scottish investigators conducted a "rapid evidence review" of the literature on institutional or residential care around the world for articles published between 2015 and 2019. The authors begin by discussing the changing and ambiguous treatment of residential care by various United Nations children's rights pronouncements. They note that those pronouncements leave a slight opening for the inclusion of residential care as their language has shifted from "institution" to "residential care." The five-year review focuses on three questions: (a) what is residential care for among the alternative forms of care?; (b) what constitutes quality in residential care?; and (c) what are the outcomes of residential care? Trying to answer these questions by only reviewing literature in a recent five-year period is problematic. However, the results of their review are surprisingly consistent with the broader perspective provided in the other four exhibits in this chapter.

The reviewers identify 111 relevant papers relevant to "institutional" or "residential" care. The papers were from 68 countries, with the largest portion from Romania and the next largest the United States. The papers represent 103 studies and eight reviews. They are not categorized by the age of residents. The reviewers encountered the problem of the unspecified independent variable. They insightfully identify the problem of distinguishing "institutional" care from "residential" care. They note that part of the difference is about size (institutions providing high child to caregiver ratios versus the lower ratios in smaller residences), but they also recognize that there are cultural differences between the two and across countries.

Giraldi et al. list as uses of residential care in the literature parent loss or respite, the failure of other forms of care, treatment or rehabilitation offered by the care site, and protection. For individual children or youth, residential care often serves multiple purposes. The question of quality is rarely central in the articles reviewed, but often is mentioned. The key aspect of quality is the caregiver-resident relationship. Effective caregivers balance warmth, sensitive affection, and playfulness with control and structure (see Chapter 6). Particularly important is a low caregiver to child ratio. The review identifies little information on outcomes based on clear comparisons of institutional or residential care to other forms of care except for studies related to the Bucharest Early Intervention Project. The authors note the

> ...continual conflation and confusion as to the nature of the setting presented, with some papers explicitly looking at institutional settings with poor care, while others looked at recognizably residential settings, and a large number did not describe the setting in any detail.
>
> (Giraldi et al., p. 831)

The results on outcomes are heavily influenced by studies on deprived settings housing infants and very young children: "...(a) substantial proportion of the papers on outcomes for children in residential care were informed by the BEIP" (p. 831).

The advantage of a rapid evidence review is that it addresses specific questions. The disadvantage is that it brings together a heterogeneous set of papers that are difficult to generalize from and Giraldi et al. were loath to try to generalize from their findings. For instance, in the unpublished report (Porter et al., 2020) they say:

> Finally, it is worth highlighting that the BEIP has had a significant impact on our understanding of institutional care on children and young people. However, the impact of the BEIP (and other studies) has been such that our expectations of residential care are significantly different from the environment experienced by the children and young people involved in the BEIP. While it is understandably frequently cited in other papers in this review, its findings are limited to the impacts of the environment in which it took place.
>
> (Porter et al., 2020, p. 42)

The narrow publishing time frame of the rapid review (a broader time period results in too many studies, hampering rapidity) also severely limits the conclusions that can be reached. That narrowness probably accounts for the tortured concluding statements in the article and the report.

Despite the narrow period covered by their review, Giraldi et al.'s findings reflect the pattern seen before in this book. First, the reviewers found few insights that could be used by policy makers to help individual children.

The reviewers were frustrated by what we called the independent variable problem in Chapter 3:

> Many of the studies analysed failed to provide definitions or descriptions of the care setting being studied or evaluated and lacked detail, for example, in the ratio between caregivers and children or the nature of the care they offered.
>
> (Giraldi et al., p. 832)

Second, little of the available literature applies to the kinds of residential care offered in the United States, Canada, the United Kingdom and elsewhere in the 21st century. In the section on "outcomes of residential care." Giraldi et al. cites 23 different published articles. Ten of those articles came from the Bucharest Early Intervention Project and another provides a review relying heavily on research from the same project. Five others deal with infants and very young children from institutions in Romania, Jordan, Ukraine, Russia, and Hungary. Those 16 papers further the long-held conclusion that early severe deprivation is a threat to development. Two papers report on small-scale studies of problems with care and adoption in Latin America. One focuses on measurement issues in studies of care in Portugal. Two others, also from Portugal, show that the quality of relationships with institutional staff and the presence of siblings are positively correlated with good outcomes in care. One study more relevant to the effectiveness of residential care compares children and youth in Rwandan orphanages with those in intact Rwandan families on measures of psychological health. Those in orphanages scored higher on the externalizing behavior scale of the Child Behavior Checklist, but there were no differences between the groups on internalizing behaviors or self-esteem.

The only other cited study in the Giraldi et al. outcomes section is Wright, Richard, Sosnowski, and Kliewer (2019). Wright et al. conducted a review of existing studies with an odd search strategy (confessed to as odd by the authors in their limitations section). They searched many databases, starting with 77,920 references and winding up with a hodgepodge of 38 papers published from 1972 to 2018 that include some evidence of "better-than-expected" outcomes of residential care. They include papers came from Asia, Africa, Europe (Norway, Portugal, Romania, Russia, Spain, and Turkey), and North America (one from Mexico and one from Birmingham, but the latter study was actually conducted in England, not Alabama). The studies are categorized as "descriptive" (17, three of which were conducted with infants or young children) relating within group individual differences or environmental differences with individual differences, or "interventions" (21, eight with infants and young children). In addition to being a tribute to the heterogeneity of research on residential care, the clear findings of the review are that close relationships between children, especially infants, and caregivers and high quality of care in general are associated with positive outcomes;

and that interventions can be and have been designed that improve the lot of those in residential care, including attachment interventions with caregivers, animal assisted therapy, encouragement of physical activity, and treatment for enuresis.

Relying on their review of the literature outside their selected period, Giraldi et al. conclude:

> As noted above, only the North America and Western European literature appears to offer some consensus and indicates that the usage of (quality) 'residential care' may allow for the provision of intensive supports in promoting recovery from trauma and in addressing social, emotional, and behavioural issues exhibited by older children in particular.
>
> (Giraldi et al., p. 832)

Third, Giraldi et al. remark on the absence of studies of what they call "non-institutional care." We do not know enough about the kinds of care offered in most homes for children and youth over the past 40 years. Finally, in an extension of the concern about detailing the nature of care as a research issue, Giraldi et al. point out the substantive lack of assessment of the quality of care provided and how it relates to differences in child outcomes. A major gap in the research literature is information on how particular environments fit particular children. Until such information is available, the reviewers argue: "... it is essential to keep an open mind as to what residential care can offer for children, in and of itself, and to understand who could most benefit from it, rather than always considering it as a measure of last resort" (Giraldi et al., 2022, p. 833).

Summary: Is Residential Care Ineffective or Harmful?

In this chapter, we reviewed five sources of evidence that counter the conventional wisdom that residential care is ineffective or even inevitably harmful for children and youth. These sources and others (e.g., Bettmann & Jasperson, 2009) show that children and youth typically do well in residential care: (a) according to retrospective self-reports, most alumni of children's homes are positive about their experiences and few of those alumni would have, retrospectively, preferred to have been in a foster family. These responses suggest that many of the American children's homes of the mid-20th century often may have been closed on a false premise, i.e., that they were ineffective; (b) the Duke Positive Outcomes for Orphans and OSCAR projects indicate that even in low-resource countries, carefully planned and executed residential care can provide positive developmental environments for young children; (c) although methodological weaknesses plague the research comparing residential care to other forms of care, it suggests that what matters most is the quality of care, not where it occurs; (d) the absence of declines and presence of almost uniform increases in the wellbeing of children and youth while they are in residential care preclude conclusions that it is inherently harmful; and (e) the most recent available research reinforces a positive view of residential care and a need for an open mind in considering it. Bad environments for children and youth need to be identified and eliminated in whatever settings they occur. However, categorically eliminating residential care as an option in the continuum of care will harm significant numbers of children and youth for whom residential care is the best fit. There is a great need for thoughtful analysis and empirical research to find for whom residential care is the best alternative. In the current anti-residential care climate, that kind of thinking and research is not likely to occur.

Lee (2020) comes to similar conclusions about effectiveness despite beginning her chapter with a defensive statement about some readers being surprised by finding a chapter on residential treatment under the heading of effective programs and practices. First, Lee concludes that the research findings on effectiveness depend on the specific characteristics of the programs being studied and what those programs are being compared with. Second, the quality of the programming rather than the site where it is administered (residential, family, foster family) matters most. Group care settings are not inherently worse than other forms of care "...and high-quality group care may produce equivalent or better outcomes than family care" (p. 308). Lee's assessment of the available research comparing residential care to alternatives, much of it reviewed in Exhibit 3 above, leads her to conclude:

> Overall outcomes favored family-based care settings with a small to medium effect size. However, when the residential program was evidence-based, there were no outcome differences between residential and family care settings, suggesting *the quality of the program influences its effectiveness.*
>
> (p. 308, my emphasis)

Third, there are dimensions of quality care that are clear. Finally, it is likely that there are interaction effects: children with different case histories and characteristics may respond to different forms of care (an obvious example is that a child who has been in a dozen different foster care placements may respond differentially to yet another foster care placement than to a high-quality residential care setting). Lee has no need to be defensive.

In Chapter 6, we will explore dimensions of quality that have been posited and supported by research.

References

Anglin, J. P., & Knorth, E. J. (2004). Competing declarations on residential care for children and youth—Stockholm versus Malmö [Editorial]. *Child and Youth Care Forum*, *33*, 141–149. doi: 10.1023/B:CCAR.0000029720.18947.66.

Axford, N., Little, M., Morpeth, L., & Weyts, A. (2005). Evaluating children's services: Recent conceptual and methodological developments. *British Journal of Social Work*, *35*, 73–88. doi:10.1093/bjsw/bch163.

Barth, R. P., Greeson, J. K. P., Guo, S., Green, R. L., Duppong Hurley, S., & Sisson, J. (2007). Outcomes for youth receiving intensive in-home therapy or residential care: A comparison using propensity scores. *American Journal of Orthopsychiatry*, *77*, 497–505. doi: 10.1037/0002-9432.77.4.497.

Bettmann, J. E., & Jasperson, R. A. (2009). Adolescents in residential and inpatient treatment: A review of the outcome literature. *Child & Youth Care Forum*, *38*, 161–183. doi: 10.1007/s10566-009-9073-y.

Bezeczky, Z., El-Banna, A., Petrou, S., Kemp, A., Scourfield, J., Forrester, D., & Nurmatov, U. B. (2020). Intensive family preservation services to prevent out-of-homeplacement of children: A systematic review and meta-analysis. *Child Abuse and Neglect*, *102*, 104394. doi: 10.1016/j.chiabu.2020.104394.

Bornstein, M. H. (2015). Children's parents. In R. M. Lerner, M. H. Bornstein, & T. Leventhal (Eds.), *Handbook of child psychology and developmental science: Ecological settings and processes* (7th ed., Vol. 4, pp. 55 132). Hoboken, NJ: Wiley. doi: 10.1002/9781118963418.childpsy403.

Byrnes, E. I., Hansen, K. G., Malloy, T. E., Carter, C., & Curry, D. (1999). Reductions in criminality subsequent to group, individual and family therapy in adolescent residential and day treatment settings. *International Journal of Group Psychotherapy*, *49*, 307–322. doi: 10.1080/00207284.1999.11732608.

Campbell, J. M. (2000). Looking back to see ahead. *Residential Treatment for Children & Youth*, *17*, 95–102. doi: 10.1300/J007v17n03_14.

Chamberlain, P., Leve, L. D., & DeGarmo, D. S. (2007). Multidimensional treatment foster care for girls in the juvenile justice system: 2-year follow-up of a randomized clinical trial. *Journal of Consulting and Clinical Psychology*, *75*, 187–193. doi: 10.1037/0022-006X.75.1.187.

Chamberlain, P., & Reid, J. B. (1998). Comparison of two community alternatives to incarceration for chronic juvenile offenders. *Journal of Consulting and Clinical Psychology*, *66*, 624–633. doi: 10.1037/0022-006X.66.4.624.

Deschenes, E. P., & Greenwood, P. W. (1998). Alternative placements for juvenile offenders: Results from the evaluation of the Nokomis Challenge Program. *Journal of Research in Crime and Delinquency*, *35*, 267–294. doi: 10.1177/0022427898035003002.

DeSena, A. D., Murphy, R. A., Douglas-Palumberi, H., Blau, G., Kelly, B., Horwitz, S. M., & Kaufman, J. (2005). SAFE Homes: Is it worth the cost? An evaluation of a group home permanency planning program for children who first enter out-of-home care. *Child Abuse & Neglect*, *29*, 627–643. doi: 10.1016/j.chiabu.2004.05.007.

Eddy, J. M., & Chamberlain, P. (2000). Family management and deviant peer association as mediators of the impact of treatment condition on youth antisocial behavior. *Journal of Consulting and Clinical Psychology*, *68*, 857–863. doi: 10.1037/0022-006X.68.5.857.

Eddy, J. M., Whaley, R. B., & Chamberlain, P. (2004). The prevention of violent behavior by chronic and serious male juvenile offenders: A 2-year follow-up of a randomized clinical trial. *Journal of Emotional and Behavioral Disorders*, *12*, 2–8. doi: 10.1177/10634266040120010101.

Embleton, L., Ayuku, D., Kamanda, A., Atwoli, L. Ayaya, S., Vreeman, R., … Braitstein, P. (2014). Models of care for orphaned and separated children and upholding children's rights: Cross-sectional evidence from western Kenya. *BMC International Health and Human Rights*, *14*(9). doi: 10.1186/1472-698X-14-9.

Fields, E., Farmer, E. M. Z., Apperson, J., Mustillo, S., & Simmers, D. (2006). Treatment and posttreatment effects of residential treatment using a Re-education Model. *Behavioral Disorders*, *31*, 312–322. doi: 10.1177/019874290603100302.

Friedrich, W. N., Baker, A. J., Parker, R., Schneiderman, M., Gries, L., & Archer, M. (2005). Youth with problematic sexualized behaviors in the child welfare system: A one-year longitudinal study. *Sexual Abuse: A Journal of Research and Treatment*, *17*, 391–406. doi: 10.1007/s11194-005-8051-7.

Ganong, L., Coleman, M., & Russell, L. T. (2015). Children in diverse families. In R. M. Lerner, M. H. Bornstein, & T. Leventhal (Eds.), *Handbook of child psychology and developmental science: Ecological settings and processes* (7th ed., Vol. 4, pp. 133–174). Hoboken, NJ: Wiley.

Gelles, R. (1999). Family preservation and child maltreatment. In R. McKenzie (Ed.), *Rethinking orphanages for the 21st century* (pp. 47–62). Thousand Oaks, CA: Sage Publications.

Giraldi, M., Mitchell, F., Porter, R. B., Reed, D., Jans, V., McIver, L., Manole, M., ... McTier, A. (2022). Residential care as an alternative care option: A review of literature within a global context. *Child & Family Social Work*, *27*, 825–837. doi: 10.1111/cfs.12929.

Gray, C. L., Pence, B. W., Ostermann, J., Whetter, R. A., O'Donnell, K., Thielman, N. M., & Whetten, K. (2015). Prevalence and incidence of traumatic experiences among orphans in institutional and family-based settings in 5 low- and middle-income countries: A longitudinal study. *Global Health: Science and Practice*, *3*, 395–404. doi: 10.9745/GHSP-D-15-00093.

Gray, C. L., Whetten, K., Messer, L. C., Whetten, R. A., Ostermann, J., O'Donnell, K., ... Pence, B. W. (2016). Potentially traumatic experiences and sexual health among orphaned and separated adolescents in five low- and middle-income countries. *Aids Care*, *28*, 857–865. doi: 10.1080/09540121.2016.1147013.

Gutterswijk, R. V., Kuiper, C. H. Z., Lautan, N., Kunst, E. G., van der Horst, F. C. P., Stams, G. J. J. M., & Prinzie, P. (2020). The outcome of non-residential youth care compared to residential youth care: A multilevel meta-analysis. *Children and Youth Services Review*, *113*, 104950. doi: 10.1016/j.childyouth.2020.104950.

Hobbs, N. (1966). Helping disturbed children: Psychological and ecological strategies. *American Psychologist*, *21*, 1105–1115. doi: 10.1037/h0021115.

Holmes, L., Connolly, C., Mortimer, E., & Hevesi, R. (2018). Residential group care as a last resort: Challenging the rhetoric. *Residential Treatment for Children & Youth*, *35*, 209–224. doi: 10.1080/0886571X.2018.1455562.

Huhr, S., & Wulczyn, F. (2022). Do intensive in-home services prevent placement?: A case study of Youth Villages' Intercept® program. *Children and Youth Services Review*, *132*, 106294. doi: 10.1016/j.childyouth.2021.106294.

Huynh H. V., Limber, S. P., Gray, C. L., Thompson, M. P., Wasonga, A. I., Vann, V., ... Whetten, K. (2019). Factors affecting the psychosocial well-being of orphan and separated children in five low- and middle-income countries: Which is more important, quality of care or care setting? *PLoS ONE*, *14*(6), e0218100. doi: 10.1371/journal.pone.0218100.

James, S. (2011). What works in group care?—A structured review of treatment models for group homes and residential care. *Children and Youth Services Review*, *33*, 308–321. doi: 10.1016/j.childyouth.2010.09.014.

Jones, M. B. (1993). Decline of the American orphanage, 1941-1980. *Social Services Review*, *67*, 459–480. doi: 10.1086/603999.

Kendrick, A. (2013). Relations, relationships and relatedness: Residential child care and the family metaphor. *Child and Family Social Work*, *18*, 77–86. doi: 10.1111/cfs.12040.

Kerr, D. C. R., Leve, L. D., & Chamberlain, P. (2009). Pregnancy rates among juvenile justice girls in two randomized controlled trials of multidimensional treatment foster care. *Journal of Consulting and Clinical Psychology*, *77*, 588–593. doi: 10.1037/a0015289.

Knorth, E. J., Harder, A. T., Zandberg, T., & Kendrick, A. J. (2008). Under one roof: A review and selective meta-analysis on the outcomes of residential child and youth care. *Children and Youth Services Review*, *30*, 123–140. doi: 10.1016/j.childyouth.2007.09.001.

Lausten, M. (2023). Residential care for children and youth in Denmark. In J. K. Whittaker, L. Holmes, J. F. del Valle, & S. James (Eds.), *Revitalizing residential care for children and youth: Cross-national trends and challenges* (pp. 225–238). New York: Oxford University Press. doi: 10.1093/oso/9780197644300.003.0016.

Lee, B. R. (2020). Residential programs: Opportunities and challenges in the 21st-century treatment environment. In T. W. Farmer, M. A. Conroy, E. M. Z. Farmer, & K. S. Sutherland (Eds.), *Handbook of research on emotional and behavioral disorders: Interdisciplinary developmental perspectives on children and youth* (pp. 306–320). New York: Routledge. doi: 10.4324/9780429453106-21.

Lee, B. R., Bright, C. L., Svoboda, D. V., Fakunmoju, S., & Barth, R. P. (2011). Outcomes of group care for youth: A review of comparative studies. *Research on Social Work Practice*, *21*, 177–189. doi: 10.1177/1049731510386243.

Lee, B. R., & Thompson, R. (2008). Comparing outcomes for youth in treatment foster care and family-style group care. *Children and Youth Services Review*, *30*, 746–757. doi: 10.1016/j.childyouth.2007.12.002.

Leve, L. D., & Chamberlain, P. (2007). A randomized evaluation of multidimensional treatment foster care: Effects on school attendance and homework completion in juvenile justice girls. *Residential Treatment for Children & Youth*, *17*, 657–663.

Leve, L. D., Chamberlain, P., & Reid, J. B. (2005). Intervention outcomes for girls referred from juvenile justice: Effects on delinquency. *Journal of Consulting and Clinical Psychology*, *73*, 1181–1185. doi: 10.1037/0022-006X.73.6.1181.

Malia, M. G., Quigley, R., Dowty, G., & Danjczek, M. (2008). The historic role of residential group care. *Reclaiming Children and Youth*, *17*, 43–51. Retrieved from: https://cyc-net.org/cyc-online/cyconline-oct2009-malia.html

Mann-Feder, V. R. (1996). Adolescents in therapeutic communities. *Adolescence*, *31*, 17–28. PMID: 9173783.

McKenzie, R. (1997). Orphanage alumni: How they have done and how they evaluate their experience. *Child & Youth Care Forum*, *26*, 87–111. doi: 10.1007/BF02589359.

McKenzie, R. B. (1996). *The Home: A memoir of growing up in an orphanage*. New York: Basic Books.

McKenzie, R. B. (Ed.). (1999). *Rethinking orphanages for the 21st century*. Thousand Oaks, CA: Sage.

McKenzie, R. B. (2003). The impact of orphanages on the alumni's lives and assessments of their childhoods. *Children and Youth Services Review*, *25*, 703–753. doi: 10.1016/S0190-7409(03)00068-9.

McKenzie, R. B. (Ed.). (2009). *Home away from home: The forgotten history of orphanages*. New York: Encounter Books.
McKenzie, R. B. (2018, November 23). The success story of orphanages. *The Weekly Standard*.
Nixon, C., & Henderson, G. (2022). How is the provision of residential care to children under the age of 12 associated with changes in children's behaviour and mental wellbeing? *Scottish Journal of Residential Child Care*, *21*(1). Retrieved from: https://strathprints.strath.ac.uk/84133/1/Nixon_Henderson_SJRCC_2022_How_is_the_provision_of_residential_care.pdf.
Porter, R. B., Giraldi, M., & Mitchell, F. (2020). *Function, quality and outcomes of residential care-rapid evidence review*. Retrieved from: https://www.celcis.org/knowledge-bank/search-bank/function-quality-and-outcomes-residential-care-rapid-evidence-review.
Portwood, S. G., Boyd, A. S., & Murdock, T. B. (2016). Implementation of a program of outcomes research in residential care settings: Outcomes for children and youth. *Child & Youth Care Forum*, *45*, 393–407. doi: 10.1007/s10566-015-9337-7.
Portwood, S. G., Boyd, S. A., Nelson, E. B., Murdock, T. B., Hamilton, J., & Miller, A. D. (2018). A comparison of outcomes for children and youth in foster and residential group care across agencies. *Children and Youth Services Review*, *85*, 19–25. doi: 10.1016/j.childyouth.2017.11.027.
Prebble, S. C., Addis, D. R., & Tippett, L. J. (2013). Autobiographical memory and sense of self. *Psychological Bulletin*, *139*, 815–840. doi: 10.1037/a0030146.
Rock, S., Michelson, D., Thomson, S., & Day, C. (2015). Understanding foster placement instability for looked after children: A systematic review and narrative synthesis of quantitative and qualitative evidence. *British Journal of Social Work*, *45*, 177–203. doi:10.1093/bjsw/bct084
Ryan, J. P., Marshall, J. M., Herz, D., & Hernandez, P. M. (2008). Juvenile delinquency in child welfare: Investigating group home effects. *Children and Youth Services Review*, *30*, 1088–1099. doi: 10.1016/j.childyouth.2008.02.004.
Schweitzer, D. D., Pecora, P. J., Nelson, K., Walters, B., & Blythe, B. J. (2015). Building the evidence base for intensive family preservation services. *Journal of Public Child Welfare*, *9*, 423–443. doi: 10.1080/15548732.2015.1090363.
Shogren, E., & Mehren, E. (1994, December 26). Close look suggests role of orphanage a complex one: Children--politicians see an easy solution, but needs of today's neglected youths are not amenable to a quick fix. *Los Angeles Times*, A1. Retrieved from: https://www.proquest.com/results/4E93BEB3DEC54BC6PQ/1?accountid=14968.
Thompson, R. W., Smith, G. L., Osgood, D. W., Dowd, T. P., Friman, G.L., & Daly, D. L. (1996). Residential care: A study of short- long-term educational effects. *Children and Youth Services Review*, *18*, 221–242. doi: 10.1016/0190-7409(96)00002-3.
Whetten, K., Ostermann, J., Pence, B. W., Whetten, R. A., Messer, L. C., Ariely, S., … The Positive Outcomes for Orphans (POFO) Research Team. (2014). Three-year change in the wellbeing of orphaned and separated children in institutional and family-based care settings in five low- and middle-income countries. *PLoS ONE*, *9*(8), e104872. doi: 10.1371/journal.pone.0104872.
Whetten, K., Ostermann, J., Whetten, R. A., Pence, B. W., O'Donnell, K., Messer, L. C., & Thielman, N. M. (2009). A comparison of the well being of orphans and abandoned children ages 6–12 in institutional and community-based care

settings in 5 less wealthy nations. *PLoS One*, *4*(12), e8169. doi: 10.1371/journal.pone.0008169.

Weinstein, L. (1969). Project Re-Ed schools for emotionally disturbed children: Effectiveness as viewed by referring agencies, parents, and teachers. *Exceptional Children*, *35*, 703–711.

Wright, A. W., Richard, S., Sosnowski, D. W., & Kliewer, W. (2019). Predictors of better functioning among institutionalized youth: A systematic review. *Journal of Child and Family Studies*, *28*, 3245–3267. doi: 10.1007/s10826-019-01527-0.

6 Do We Know What Quality Residential Care Is?

The conventional wisdom about residential care is wrong, but that does not mean that just any kind of care will do. Children and youth in care deserve the highest quality care possible, regardless of its monetary cost. That is especially true for those who have been harmed by their families and society. There are clear indications that the quality of care is more important than the site of the care in the literature already reviewed. As Holmes, Connolly, Mortimer, and Hevesi (2018) summarize:

> Studies within the field of child welfare show that it is not the individual versus group nature of the care environment but rather it is the quality of the care provided that affects outcomes.
>
> (p. 215)

That makes sense if resources and stability are the greatest factors in developmental outcomes. Because quality of care is so important, we must be careful to discern those components of quality that enhance physical, cognitive, and social-emotional development. Just what resources are required and how can stability be maintained?

Some scholars and pundits have argued that quality childcare, particularly residential childcare, is impossible to define or that we would not know it if we saw it. I believe that to be untrue. Others argue that unless we can test versions of care in rigorous, evidence-based, randomized clinical trials, we will not know what quality care is. Originally used in medicine (Sackett & Rosenberg, 1995), the term "evidence-based" is now used in many disciplines, including psychotherapy (Lilienfeld, 2019) and social work (Gibbs & Gambrill, 2002). The term is usually used as shorthand for "scientific" or "objective," terms with their own philosophical problems. However, all evidence must be contextualized and interpreted. The "evidence" in evidence-based can be results of randomized clinical trials, quasi-experiments, field studies, case studies, and even expert clinical observations (see the summary of James, 2011, in Chapter 5). Rarely is just one side of a social science argument supported by evidence. Judgment about the validity and applicability

DOI: 10.4324/9781003435709-6

of the "evidence" will always require a degree of wise discernment. Perhaps what fits "evidence-based" in the study of residential care is something like what the journalist Carl Bernstein has called "the best obtainable version of the truth." I would add "at this time." We need a substantial dose of humility with our judgments about quality care. The history of care for children is one in which we thought we knew what is best until we find out that we did not.

I think a purely "evidence-based" form of childcare is an illusion. There will always be legitimate debates about what constitutes best evidence. The point of Chapter 3 was to warn readers of the residential care literature about facile interpretations of evidence. Indeed, the heart of this book is a claim that evidence has been misinterpreted and misapplied. Therefore, in this chapter, I argue that with clinical judgment based on child development theory, bits and pieces of empirical research, and a dose of common sense, we can describe high-quality residential care. We can do so in a way that we can see it, know it, use it, assess it, and disseminate it. But I do so without claiming the vaunted descriptor "evidence-based." The reader will have to settle for "evidence-informed."

In some ways high-quality residential care looks like other forms of quality child care. However, the mixture of special needs and unusual life histories of children in care precludes simple generalizations. There is great variation in existing residential care, centering on dimensions of child and youth autonomy, caregiver and peer relations, safety and security, and support for transitions to adulthood (Cameron-Mathiassen, Leiper, Simpson, & McDermott, 2022). What we already know about what works in residential care is a good start. In the United Kingdom, some scholars argue that it is possible to differentiate residences that produce good and poor outcomes (Clough, 2005). Residential care can provide a good place to live, not a fallback when all else fails. Not something to be prevented, but an important part of an array of potential services for children and youth. What is presented here is not a manual of operations. It is a continuation of efforts toward defining good practice. It is consistent with other attempts to describe high-quality residential care (a good example is Smith, 2009).

What Do Children and Youth Need?

General reviews of the literature in child psychology (e.g., see Ganong, Coleman, & Russell, 2015 specifically and other chapters on parenting and families in the various editions of the *Handbook of Child Psychology*) suggest that children and youth need two things for optimal chances development: resources and stability. Perhaps that is oversimplified, but when accounting for differences in child outcomes, these broad categories explain a lot. Defining and assessing quality of care requires attention to both. The resources children need in their physical and social environments are not necessarily linearly related to outcomes. It may not be a matter of "more is better," especially in the realm of physical resources. There may be optimal levels of resources in the middle range of physical assets and social relationships. For example, stimulation from physical objects is important but children and youth can be overstimulated. Neither extreme poverty nor extreme wealth optimize development (Luthar & Barkin, 2012). Social relationships also can be "too much" when they are too many or too intrusive. Moreover, physical and social resources are not independent. The physical world is mediated by the social in many ways (Bronfenbrenner & Ceci, 1994). Inert resources rarely influence development.

We will look at the quality of residential care resources in two ways. First, we will use Maslow's well-known motivation hierarchy to look at basic resources. Second, we will look at resources in more detail using the ecological framework of Urie Bronfenbrenner (1979; Bronfenbrenner & Morris, 2006). His nested systems approach is particularly applicable to the resources offered (or not) by residential care. In applying these views, it is important to keep two major qualifications in mind. First, we are talking about resources for children five years of age and above (see Chapter 4). Second, the direct unit of care must be small. It is unlikely that high-quality residential care can be offered to more than six to ten children or youth at a time or by more than two different sets of caregivers in seven to ten day alternating periods (Knorth, Harder, Zandberg, & Kendrick, 2008; Osei & Gorey, 2019; Roca, Garcia, Biarne, & Rodriguez, 2009).

The question of resources is relatively straightforward. The concept of stability offers more challenges. One aspect of stability is change or transitions in physical and social environments. Stability also reflects predictability, continuity, and degrees of permanence. For children and youth, stability may most clearly be measured by the degree to which physical resources in Bronfenbrenner's systems change over time ("home," school, neighborhood, peer group). After his initial 1979 conceptualization, Bronfenbrenner added a time dimension, the "chronosystem." The child welfare system in many countries has failed significant numbers of children and youth over time by not providing stable physical and social resources (for illustrative firsthand accounts from the United States, see Brown & Seita, 2009). The concept of "least restrictive environment" has dominated how the environments of vulnerable children and youth have been judged over that past 60 years. A search for less restrictive caregiving structures (without a clear definition of "restrictive") often influences decisions about placement with little regard to stability, continuity, and predictability in the child's experience. The family of biological origin is seen as the least restrictive environment for care with approximations (especially foster care) to that form of care judged to be less restrictive and thus of higher quality than residential care. Multiple trials (placements) in a less restrictive environment are seen as superior to fewer changes in what are deemed as more restrictive settings (Konijn et al., 2019). The evidence on the number of placements foster children experience suggests that the trade-off between restrictiveness and stability is not always a good one (e.g., Chambers et al., 2018).

Children need psychological stability, not just stability in physical and social resources. Children organize their experiences with mental models that cognitive psychologists call "schemas" or "scripts" and attachment theorists call "working models" (Bretherton & Munholland, 2008). The idea of working models reflects the child's ongoing revisioning of their models in response to their changing physical and social experiences. Individuals construct working models of many aspects of their experience. Attachment theorists stress the fundamental working model infants and toddlers have based on their interactions with caregivers and the degree to which caregivers respond in a sensitive way to their signals of need. During development, children develop working models of "family," "home," "school," "friendship," "self," and many other components of their experience in response to positive and negative feedback.

As children develop, their various working models and the relationships among those working models change in complex ways. For children and youth in out-of-home care, the working models surrounding family, adult-child relations, friendships, school, and their interrelationships can be particularly complex and fragile. Frequent changes in their environments can make for substantial instability and ego brittleness (using "ego brittleness" as the opposite of "ego resiliency" or adaptiveness in Block's sense, Block & Kremen, 1996). Ultimately, one major indicator of the quality of residential care is how well it provides stability, not only in physical and social resources, but provides for psychological stability.

Quality of Residential Care: A Hierarchy of Needs Perspective

There is good reason that Abraham Maslow's hierarchy of needs is one of the most popular and popularized ideas in psychology (Maslow, 1943). It taps into basic truths about human motivation. Maslow's pyramid illustrates how some motivational systems at the lower level are more basic to survival whereas others at higher levels reflect greater degrees of developmental adaptation. The lesson for high-quality residential care is that there can be no compromise about meeting the needs of children and youth at the most basic levels. Adequate provisions must be made for nutritional and health care (Huynh, 2019; Nelson et al., 2013) and residents must be safe, free from any kind of staff or peer abuse (Farmer, Murray, Ballentine, Rauktis, & Burns, 2017; Hermenau, Goessman, Rygaard, Landolt, & Hecker, 2017; Huynh, 2019; Moore, McArthur, Death, Tilbury, & Roche, 2017). Moreover, residents must *feel* safe (Nijhof, Veerman, Engels, & Scholte, 2011; Slaatto, Kleppe, Mellblom, & Baugerud, 2023). For those children and youth in residential care because of abuse or neglect, "family" has not been a safe place (as one of Moore et al.'s (2017) respondents said about his residential care site, "it's got to be better than home"). There will be some detail on Maslow's next highest, "relationship" level in the next section. It is the heart of high-quality residential care. Neagu (2021) summarizes it nicely:

> ...children in care want to feel loved, safe, respected; they want to have their say in how they are cared for, not to be separated from siblings as they enter care; they want to have a sense of who they are, to be able to maintain positive relationships; they want to know what their rights are.
> (Neagu, 2021, p. 49)

There can be no real quality if the residential institution cannot provide rich caregiver-resident reciprocal relationships. However, it is at the peak of Maslow's pyramid where the highest quality residential programs will distinguish themselves. The best programs will help residents gain self-esteem and even self-actualize as they set meaningful goals and gain competence in multiple domains (Strijbosch et al., 2014). Those programs will stimulate curiosity and exploration using developmentally important challenges in and out of formal educational settings (Anthony, Krysik, & Kelly, 2019; Holden, 2009; Huynh, 2019; Strijbosch et al., 2014; Sulimani-Aidan, 2018).

Maslow's scheme provides a general structure for thinking about high-quality care, but it is not specific enough to give residential programs clear guidelines. In the next section, we will look at the kind of program characteristics that can begin to operationalize high quality.

An Ecological Perspective on High-quality Residential Care

Urie Bronfenbrenner's approach to modeling environment-child relations (1979) is a useful framework for considering high-quality residential care. It is useful because it provides both a comprehensive catalog of the parts of the residential life directly affected by aspects of the environment and a means of thinking about the wider implications of the organizational and policy realms for residential programming. The framework used here is based on Bronfenbrenner's original ecological theory. The later version of his theory (Bronfenbrenner & Evans, 2000) will be discussed as it relates to the CARE model of residential care in Chapter 7.

Microsystem components. In Bronfenbrenner's original version, the environment is modeled as concentric circles of influence. The most direct, day to day, influences are in microsystems. They include family/parents/caregivers, school, peer groups, playgrounds, clinics, and other people and spaces children frequent regularly. The determination of the quality of residential care depends greatly on what goes on in the component microsystems. In the **caregiver microsystem**, the caregivers are not parents (although in many organizations they are called "house parents" and have been so for decades), but many of the indicators of quality are the same. They are the ones who are with the children or youth on a regular, predictable schedule

(Farmer et al., 2017; Sekol, 2013). Although the attainment of a secure caregiver relationship is normally a task for infants and toddlers (Ainsworth, Blehar, Waters, & Wall, 1978), many children in residential care have never formed a secure attachment to any caregiver (Hermenau et al., 2017). High-quality residential care needs to provide the secure base that children and youth can use to explore their environments and develop a sense of safety they may have never experienced (Anglin & Scott, 2019). Caregivers who consistently respond to the resident's emotional signals can help build a child's internal working model of a caretaker as one who offers a feeling of predictability and normality (Ward, 2004). In residential care this sense of normality may result from many small things like the deinstitutionalized hominess of the campus, enriched celebrations of holidays and birthdays, special trips, and rewards and recognition for achievements and good behavior. In high-quality residential care, caregivers act as teachers, mentors, coaches, sympathizers, defenders, and advocates (Anglin, 2004; Anglin & Scott, 2019). The adults in high-quality residential care follow a modified golden rule: treat residents as you would want your own children to be treated (indeed, on many residential care campuses, the children of caregivers live with the residents when their parents are on duty). Although the research on size and outcomes is not completely clear (e.g., Chipenda-Dansokho & Bullock, 2003), the adult-child ratio of 2/6–10 that has become normative in children's homes is probably reasonable to meet the microsystem characteristics listed here.

Adult-child/youth interactions in high-quality residential care are the same as those that characterize good parents in other family structures (Anglin, 2004; Huynh, 2019). Adult caregivers need to communicate availability, consistency, and unconditional positive regard (Kelly, Anthony, & Krysik, 2019; McCrea & Bulanda, 2010) and be emotionally warm, supportive, and responsive (Sulimani-Aidan, 2018). Structure and discipline are important with rules that are fair (Moore et al., 2017), consistently enforced, and negotiated over time through give and take (Aussems, Muntinga, Addink, & Dedding, 2020; Rauktis, Fusco, Cahalane, Bennett, & Reinhart, 2011). Residents want staff to "try to make it seem we're regular kids" (Rauktis et al., 2011). Consistent with the highest level of Maslow's hierarchy, the adults in high-quality residential care have high, developmentally appropriate expectations for residents (Beker, 2001), challenging residents to do better (Holden, 2009; Palareti & Berti, 2009; Ward, 2004) but making sure there is room for error (Aussems et al., 2020). In high-quality residential care, children and youth are seen as "at promise," not "at risk" (Anglin, 2004; Anglin & Scott, 2019). Caregivers who are low in warmth, who are punitive and authoritarian, who are permissive, who harbor low expectations, who cannot communicate, are not capable of delivering high-quality residential care (Bastiaanssen et al., 2014).

For children and youth who have moved from placement to placement, the **school/education microsystem** is crucial. Frequent changes in schools are related to lower achievement (Mehana & Reynolds, 2004; Olsen & de Montgomery, 2018). Whether their day-to-day education takes place on- or off-campus, most residents will need educational supplements. This may come in the form of tutoring (Forsman, 2020; Zeller & Köngeter, 2012), educational advising, and counseling (Del Quest et al., 2012; Huefner, 2018; Huynh, 2019; Ringle, Ingram, & Thompson, 2010). Because of their residents' checkered educational pasts, it is particularly important for caregivers and teachers to have what Carol Dweck has called an "incremental" or "growth" mindset about residents' learning and encourage that mindset in the residents themselves (Yeager & Dweck, 2012). In contrast to learners with a "trait" or "fixed" mindset, learners with incremental mindsets believe that failure is not an indication of a lack of inherent ability, but information to be used to make greater or different, more productive efforts. Caregivers and teachers who have an incremental mindset do not give up on learners, believing they have reached the limits of their ability. Instead, they look for new and better ways to facilitate learning. One of the major advantages of stability in residents' lives is continuity in schooling. Long-term educational success is associated with longer periods of time in residence (Thompson et al., 1996).

The microsystem perhaps next in importance to caregivers is the **peer microsystem.** One of the models for residential care examined by James (2011—see Chapter 5) is "Positive Peer Culture." That model is based on the well-supported supposition that peers have a powerful influence on each other, increasingly so during adolescence (Furman & Rose, 2015). Whether or not a peer focus can carry the weight of a comprehensive model of residential care (see the next chapter), high-quality residential care aims to develop supportive peer groups and eliminate aggression and bullying (Sekol, 2013). High-quality residential sites that serve older adolescents and young adults should have a **transitional and independent living microsystem.** It will include specific housing and program provisions for teaching life skills, providing continuing educational and vocational training opportunities, help in obtaining initial employment, and, when appropriate, opportunities for exploring family reunification (Doucet, Greeson, & Eldeeb, 2022).

There are many **other possible microsystems** in residential care. In faith-based organizations, church or other spiritual settings engage much of the residents' time. High-quality residential care will provide therapy or counseling, opportunities for community engagement through service activities, job opportunities for older youth, involvement in athletics and other extracurricular activities, and so on. For children and youth in residential care, another microsystem may be their family of origin, if they have remained connected to it. The ultimate impact of all the microsystems will depend largely on what happens at the mesosystem level.

Mesosystem. The effectiveness of residential care will depend on the quality of the microsystems, but also on how well interventions are planned at the mesosystem level so as to coordinate and integrate daily living, peer-involved activities, education, etc. (Huefner, 2018; Palareti & Berti, 2009).

For residential care, the mesosystem connections are tighter than usual. On a residential campus, children and youth live with caregivers but the campus is also their neighborhood where they play with peers, participate in organized recreation, engage in therapeutic interventions, and may even go to school and church. It is important therefore that all these components be closely coordinated (Forsman, 2020; Garcia-Molsosa, Collet-Sabé, Martoria, & Montserrat, 2019; Huefner, 2018; Knorth et al., 2008). A potential disadvantage of this tightness is that the lives of residents can be insulated and their experiences parochial. Organizations must self-consciously involve residents in the larger community to avoid narrowing the overall experience. Residential caregivers are knowledgeable about the various aspects of the resident's life and work to see that they coordinate to the resident's benefit. Peer and school interactions are more closely integrated with "family" functions and can be monitored more closely. The result can contribute to the stability and continuity for those whose pasts have so often been defined by disruption, transition, and chaos. Anglin (2002) argues that the philosophical and practice orientations of managers permeate care organizations. Selecting good leadership and avoiding turnover are keys to quality.

High-quality residential care will provide individualized plans for residents that build on their strengths. Those plans will be informed by their prior experiences, involve the children or youth (especially those who are older), and set measurable and attainable developmental, educational, vocational, and personal goals (Huynh, 2019). Two mesosystem-level connections are especially important, the ones between the caregiver and the family of origin microsystems and between the caregiver and school microsystems. Research with children and youth in psychiatric care (Attar-Schwartz, 2019; Robst, Rohrer, Dollard, & Armstrong, 2014) indicates that the chance of long-term therapeutic success increases when close contact is maintained with the resident's family. When not prohibited by courts or child welfare agencies, families should be involved in treatment decisions, there should be home visits as appropriate, and other means of maintaining contact should be employed.

Likewise, close connections should be established between caregivers and school personnel, including teachers, counselors, and administrators (Garcia-Molosa et al., 2019). Teachers need to know that caregivers value communication, children and youth should work with teachers and caretakers on their own goals, and caregivers should closely monitor the educational and behavioral progress of residents. Tutoring, counseling, and other support services available at the children's home should be closely coordinated with schools.

Exosystem. Perhaps the three most important questions about quality at the exosystem level are about how the physical environment is designed, the program or model being used, and how staff members are selected and trained. As indicated above, the direct care unit for children and youth should be a small, family-like environment of no more than six to ten children or youth, ages six or over. Whenever possible, sibling groups should be kept together (Knorth et al., 2008; Leichtentritt, 2013; Mota & Matos, 2015; Osei & Gorey, 2019). Although the notion of least restrictive environment needs to be balanced with safety, residents should have developmentally appropriate levels of freedom within the campus and also have their own space for privacy and personal possessions that allow a differentiated identity. The campus should provide ample opportunity for recreation and the pursuit of interests and hobbies. High-quality residential care campuses will be clean and attractive.

There will be closer attention to specific models of care in the next chapter, but there are some general characteristics of programs that would constitute quality care. The program will be based on a combination of research evidence, child development theory, and ethical principles for dealing with children and youth (Ward, 2004). An array of services provides for individual and developmental differences, capable of interventions that meet resident needs. Medical and counseling services are available as needed. Administrators without direct daily contact should still know residents, their histories, and their current status. Part of the programming needs to be about life after the program (Refaeli, Benbenishty, & Eliel-Gev, 2013; Robinson et al., 2012; Sulimani-Aidan & Benbenishty, 2011; Urban, Jordan, Kisiel, & Fehrenbach, 2019).

The staff members in high-quality residential care will be selected and trained carefully. Selection criteria should include the characteristics of the caregiving microsystem (warmth, high expectations, communication skills, etc.). Staff should be energetic and committed (Ward, 2004). It is obvious that staff, especially direct care staff, need to be well-trained (Hermenau et al., 2017), but there is little hard research on training for residential care (Eenshuistra, Harder, & Knorth, 2019; Roy, Marizot, Lamothe, & Geoffrion, 2020). Extensive staff training is a characteristic of the two model programs described in Chapter 7. In addition to training in the model the organization is using, staff need to learn appropriate methods of restraint and crisis management, and self-harm prevention (Crosland et al., 2008). Compensation and working conditions should be designed to discourage turnover. Staff members need regular opportunities to be heard about their work and their charges. Staff members should have regular and frequent chances to meet with each other and receive informed supervision (Reznikovski-Kuras & Gerasimenko, 2020). Continuing education should be frequent and relevant. Staff members should be centrally involved in quality improvement procedures. A particularly important issue is the smooth handoff between caregiver cycles with enough overlap that those taking over have ample opportunity to know with residents' behavioral and educational statuses. Staff members should have access to their own methods for dealing with stress (Proeschold-Bell et al., 2019).

Macrosystem. At the broadest environmental level, residential care exists in different forms in different countries and cultures (Ibrahim & Howe, 2011; Meichsner, 2021) in response to different political and economic ideologies.

There are probably some universal characteristics of high-quality care, including the establishment of attachment bonds that provide for safety and security and the transmission of the culture's norms, skills, and knowledge (Mesman & Emmen, 2021). However, even those universals will differ in form and content across cultures (Kromhout, Eldering, & Knorth, 2000). The Duke Positive Outcomes for Orphans and OSCAR projects reviewed in Chapter 5 demonstrate that high-quality residential care can be adapted to culture. Regardless, generalizations across cultures should be made cautiously.

Summary: Quality Care as Resilience Promotion

There are interesting parallels between the characteristics of high-quality residential care and those factors that promote resilience in children (Frensch, Ashbourne, MacLeod, Bartlett, & Preyde, 2022). Resilience has been treated as an individual difference dimension in personality (Block & Kremen, 1996) and as an outcome of developmental systems working together to result in successful adaptations to adversity, what Masten (2014) calls "ordinary magic." The development systems that work together include attachment, mastery motivation/self-efficacy, self-regulation (impulse control), and cognitive development (in response to education and intellectual stimulation). Resilient children develop protective adaptive skills in families from good parenting, social networks and friendships, supportive schooling, adequate health care, and well-functioning neighborhoods (Katisi et al., 2019; Mantovani, Gillard, Mezey & Clare, 2020; Racine, Eirich, & Madigan, 2022).

High-quality residential care offers children and youth equivalents to what is offered by strong parenting, strong schools, and strong neighborhoods, features often missing in their prior experience. At its best, high-quality residential care provides caregivers who develop strong attachments and a secure base for residents, authoritative interactions that encourage self-regulation and impulse control, and stable relationships with adults and peers, all aspects of an environment that research shows promote resiliency (Cameron-Mathiassen et al., 2022; Harder, Knorth, & Kalverboer, 2012; Lou, Taylor, & Di Folco, 2018; Yoon et al., 2021). Moreover, high-quality residential care offers an environment where residents can develop friendships, crime is low or nonexistent, and school engagement is enhanced, factors that promote resiliency (Hawkins-Rodgers, 2007). For children and youth who have often struggled in school, the development of educational interests and commitments that promote educational resiliency are especially important (Nuñez, Beal, & Jacquez, 2022). Sameroff and Rosenblum (2006) suggest that the child's context may be an even better predictor of competence than personal resilience. And that may be particularly true of children in residential care.

In an interesting contrast to America's "Family First," recent reforms in Denmark, where the utilization rate of residential care is triple that of the

United States, are characterized as "Children First" (Lausten, 2023). Included are emphases on: (a) earlier and better interventions; (b) stability; (c) quality; (d) children's inputs about their placements; and (e) improvements in transition and aftercare services. Those components capture the essentials of quality care anywhere. We need to know more about what constitutes quality residential care. Yet we know enough already to be able to provide quality care to the children being served today. In the next chapter, we will look in detail at two strong models of high-quality residential care.

References

Ainsworth, M. D. S., Blehar, M. C., Waters, E., & Wall, S. (1978). *Patterns of attachment: A psychological study of the strange situation*. Hillsdale, NJ: Erlbaum.

Anglin, J. P. (2002). *Pain, normality, and the struggle for congruence: Reinterpreting residential care for children and youth*. New York: Haworth Press.

Anglin, J. P. (2004). Creating "well-functioning" residential care and defining its place in a system of care. *Child & Youth Care Forum*, *33*, 175–192. doi: 10.1023/B:CCAR.0000029689.70611.0f.

Anglin, J. P., & Scott, A. (2019). Researching pain—Re-searching the researcher: Pulling back the curtain on the inner life and anxiety of the investigator. *International Journal of Child, Youth and Family Studies*, *10*(2–3), 142–155. doi: 10.18357/ijcyfs102-3201918857.

Anthony, E. K., Krysik, J., & Kelly, C. (2019). Social-emotional well-being among youth living in out-of-home care. *Children and Youth Services Review*, *96*, 381–385. doi: 10.1016/j.childyouth.2018.12.007.

Attar-Schwartz, S. (2019). Parental availability of support and frequency of contact: The reports of youth in educational residential care. *Children and Youth Services Review*, *101*, 317–328. doi: 10.1016/j.childyouth.2019.04.016.

Aussems, K., Muntinga, M., Addink, A., & Dedding, C. (2020). "Call us by our name": Quality of care and wellbeing from the perspective of girls in residential care facilities who are commercially and sexually exploited by "loverboys." *Children and Youth Services Review*, *116*, 105213. doi: 10.1016/j.childyouth.2020.105213.

Bastiaanssen, I. L. W., Delsing, M. J. M. H., Geijsen, L., Kroes, G., Veerman, J. W., & Engels, R. C. M. E. (2014). Observations of group care worker-child interaction in residential youth care: Pedagogical interventions and child behavior. *Child & Youth Care Forum*, *43*, 227–241. doi: 10.1007/s10566-013-9231-0.

Beker, J. (2001). Back to the future: Effective residential group care and treatment for children and youth and the Fritz Redl Legacy. *Child & Youth Care Forum*, *30*, 443–455. doi: 10.1023/A:1015329501206.

Block, J., & Kremen, A. M. (1996). IQ and ego-resiliency: Conceptual and empirical connections and separateness. *Journal of Personality and Social Psychology*, *70*, 349–361. doi: 10.1037/0022-3514.70.2.349.

Bretherton, I., & Munholland, K. A. (2008). Internal working models in attachment relationships: Elaborating a central construct in attachment theory. In J. Cassidy & P. R. Shaver (Eds.), *Handbook of attachment: Theory, research, and clinical applications* (pp. 102–127). New York: Guilford Press.

Bronfenbrenner, U. (1979). *The ecology of human development: Experiments by nature and design*. Cambridge, MA: Harvard University Press.

Bronfenbrenner, U., & Ceci, S. J. (1994). Nature-nurture reconceptualized in developmental perspective: A bioecological model. *Psychological Review*, *101*, 568–586. doi: 10.1037/0033-295X.101.4.568.

Bronfenbrenner, U., & Evans, G. W. (2000). Developmental science in the 21st century: Emerging questions, theoretical models, research designs and empirical findings. *Social Development*, *9*, 115–125. doi: 10.1111/1467-9507.00114.

Bronfenbrenner, U., & Morris, P. (2006). The bioecological model of human development. In R. M. Lerner & W. Damon (Eds.), *Handbook of child psychology: Theoretical models of human development* (6th ed., Vol. 1, pp. 793–828). Hoboken, NJ: Wiley.

Brown, W. K., & Seita, J. R. (Eds.). (2009). *Growing up in the care of strangers: The experiences, insights and recommendations of eleven former foster kids*. Tallahassee, FL: William Gladden Foundation Press.

Cameron-Mathiassen, J., Leiper, J., Simpson, J., & McDermott, E. (2022). What was care like for me? A systematic review of the experiences of young people living in residential care. *Children and Youth Services Review*, *138*, 106524. doi: 10.1016/j.childyouth.2022.106524.

Chambers, R. M., Crutchfield, R. M., Willis, T. Y., Cuza, H. A., Otero, A., Goddu Harper, S. G., & Carmichael, H. (2018). "It's just not right to move a kid that many times": A qualitative study of how foster care alumni perceive placement moves. *Children and Youth Services Review*, *86*, 76–83. doi: 10.1016/j.childyouth.2018.01.028.

Chipenda-Dansokho, S., & Bullock, R. (2003). The determinants and influence of size on residential settings for children. *International Journal of Child and Family Welfare*, *3*, 66–76. Retrieved from: https://ugp.rug.nl/IJCFW/article/view/37623.

Clough, R. (2005). Children in residence. In N. Axford, V. Berry, M. Little, & L. Morpeth (Eds.), *Forty years of research, policy and practice in children's services: A festschrift for Roger Bullock* (pp. 43–55). Oxford: Wiley-Blackwell.

Crosland, K. A., Dunlap, G., Sager, W., Neff, B., Wilcox, C., Blanco, A., & Giddings, T. (2008). The effects of staff training on the types of interactions observed at two group homes for foster care children. *Research on Social Work Practice*, *18*, 410–420. doi: 10.1177/1049731507314000.

Del Quest, A., Fullerton, A., Geenen, S., Powers, L., & The Research Consortium to Increase the Success of Youth in Foster Care. (2012). Voices of youth in foster care and special education regarding their educational experiences and transition to adulthood. *Children and Youth Services Review*, *34*, 1604–1615. doi: 10.1016/j.childyouth.2012.04.018.

Doucet, M. M., Greeson, J. K. P., & Eldeeb, N. (2022). Independent living programs and services for youth 'aging out' of care in Canada and the U. S.: A systematic review. *Children and Youth Services Review*, *142*, 106630. doi: 10.1016/j.childyouth.2022.106630.

Eenshuistra, A., Harder, A. T., & Knorth, E. J. (2019). One size does not fit all: A systematic review of training outcomes on residential youth care professionals' skills. *Children and Youth Services Review*, *103*, 135–147. doi: 10.1016/j.childyouth.2019.05.010.

Farmer, E. M. Z., Murray, M., Ballentine, K., Rauktis, M. E., & Burns, B. J. (2017). Would we know it if we saw it?: Assessing quality of care in group homes for youth. *Journal of Emotional and Behavioral Disorders*, *25*, 28–36. doi: 10.1177/1063426616687363.

Forsman, H. (2020). Exploring educational pathways over the life course in children with out-of-homecare experience: A multi-group path analysis. *Children and Youth Services Review, 111*, 104852. doi: 10.1016/j.childyouth.2020.104852.

Frensch, K., Ashbourne, G., MacLeod, K., Bartlett, D., & Preyde, M. (2022). Better than expected: Young adults' perceptions of community living after children's residential mental health treatment. *Residential Treatment for Children & Youth, 39*, 57–80. doi: 10.1080/0886571X.2020.1751019.

Furman, W., & Rose, A. J. (2015). Friendships, romantic relationships, and peer relationships. In R. M. Lerner & M. E. Lamb (Eds.), *Handbook of child psychology and developmental science: Socioemotional processes* (7th ed., Vol. 3). *Wiley Developmental Science in the 21st Century: Emerging Questions, Theoretical Models, Research Designs and Empirical Findings* (pp. 932–974). Hoboken, NJ: Wiley.

Ganong, L., Coleman, M., & Russell, L. T. (2015). Children in diverse families. In R. M. Lerner, M. H. Bornstein, & T. Leventhal (Eds.), *Handbook of child psychology and developmental science: Ecological settings and processes* (7th ed., Vol. 4, pp. 133–174). Hoboken, NJ: Wiley.

Garcia-Molsosa, M., Collet-Sabé, J., Martoria, J. C., & Montserrat, C. (2019). School satisfaction among youth in residential care: A multi-source analysis. *Children and Youth Services Review, 105*, 104409. doi: 10.1016/j.childyouth.2019.104409.

Gibbs, L., & Gambrill, E. (2002). Evidence-based practice: Counterarguments to objections. *Research On Social Work Practice, 12*, 452–476. doi:10.1177/1049731502012003007Harder, A. T., Knorth, E. J., & Kalverboer, M. E. (2012). A secure base? The adolescent-staff relationship in secure residential youth care. *Child and Family Social Work, 18*, 305–317. doi: 10.1111/j.1365-2206.2012.00846.x.

Hawkins-Rodgers, Y. (2007). Adolescents adjusting to a group home environment: A residential care model of re-organizing attachment behavior and building resiliency. *Children and Youth Services Review, 29*, 1131–1141. doi: 10.1016/j.childyouth.2007.04.007.

Hermenau, K., Goessmann, K., Rygaard, N. P., Landolt, M. A., & Hecker, T. (2017). Fostering child development by improving care quality: A systematic review of the effectiveness of structural interventions and caregiver trainings in institutional care. *Trauma, Violence, & Abuse, 18*, 544–561. doi: 10.1177/1524838016641918.

Holden, M. J. (2009). *Children and residential experiences: Creating conditions for change*. Arlington, VA: Child Welfare League of America.

Holmes, L., Connolly, C., Mortimer, E., & Hevesi, R. (2018). Residential group care as a last resort: Challenging the rhetoric. *Residential Treatment for Children & Youth, 35*, 209–224. doi: 10.1080/0886571X.2018.1455562.

Huefner, J. C. (2018). Crosswalk of published quality standards for residential care for children and adolescents. *Children and Youth Services Review, 88*, 267–273. doi: 10.1016/j.childyouth.2018.03.022.

Huynh, H. V. (2019). Lessons learned from high-quality residential care centers around the world: A visual story. *International Journal on Child Maltreatment: Research, Policy and Practice*, 2, 99–116. doi: 10.1007/s42448-019-00018-5.

Ibrahim, R. W., & Howe, D. (2011). The experience of Jordanian care leavers making the transition from residential care to adulthood: The influence of a patriarchal and collectivist culture. *Children and Youth Services Review, 33*, 2469–2474. doi: 10.1016/j.childyouth.2011.08.019.

James, S. (2011). What works in group care?—A structured review of treatment models for group homes and residential care. *Children and Youth Services Review*, *33*, 308–321. doi: 10.1016/j.childyouth.2010.09.014.

Katisi, M., Jeffries, P., Dikolobe, O., Moeti, O., Brisson, J., & Ungar, M. (2019). Fostering resilience in children who have been orphaned: Preliminary results from the Botswana Balekane EARTH Program. *Child & Youth Care Forum*, *48*, 585–601. doi: 10.1007/s10566-019-09497-6.

Kelly, C. Anthony, E. K., & Krysik, J. (2019). "How am I doing?" narratives of youth living in congregate care on their social-emotional well-being. *Children and Youth Services Review*, *103*, 255–263. doi: 10.1016/j.childyouth.2019.06.001.

Knorth, E. J., Harder, A. T., Zandberg, T., & Kendrick, A. J. (2008). Under one roof: A review and selective meta-analysis on the outcomes of residential child and youth care. *Children and Youth Services Review*, *30*, 123–140. doi: 10.1016/j.childyouth.2007.09.001.

Konijn, C., Admiraal, S., Baart, J., van Rooij, F., Stams, G. J., Colonnesi, C., … Assink, M. (2019). Foster care placement instability: A meta-analytic review. *Children and Youth Services Review*, *96*, 483–499. doi: 10.1016/j.childyouth.2018.12.002.

Kromhout, M., Eldering, L., & Knorth, E. J. (2000). Cultural differences in residential child and youth care: Analyzing perspectives. *Child & Youth Care Forum*, *29*, 359–372. doi: 10.1023/A:1016697301636.

Lausten, M. (2023). Residential care for children and youth in Denmark. In J. K. Whittaker, L. Holmes, J. F. del Valle, & S. James (Eds.), *Revitalizing residential care for children and youth: Cross-national trends and challenges* (pp. 225–238). New York: Oxford University Press. doi: 10.1093/oso/9780197644300.003.0016.

Leichtentritt, J. (2013). "It is difficult to be here with my sister but intolerable to be without her": Intact sibling placement in residential care. *Children and Youth Services Review*, *35*, 762–770. doi: 10.1016/j.childyouth.2013.01.022.

Lilienfeld, S. O. (2019). What is "evidence" in psychotherapies? *World Psychiatry*, *18*, 245–246. doi: 10.1002/wps.20654.

Lou, Y., Taylor, E. P., & Di Folco, S. (2018). Resilience and resilience factors in children in residential care: A systematic review. *Children and Youth Services Review*, *89*, 83–92. doi: 10.1016/j.childyouth.2018.04.010.

Luthar, S. S., & Barkin, S. H. (2012). Are affluent youth truly "at risk"? Vulnerability and resilience across three diverse samples. *Development and Psychopathology*, *24*, 429–449. doi: 10.1017/S0954579412000089.

Mantovani, N., Gillard, S., Mezey, G., & Clare, F. (2020). Children and young people "in care" participating in a peer-mentoring relationship: An exploration of resilience. *Journal of Research on Adolescence*, *30*, S2, 380–390. doi: 10.1111/jora.12483.

Maslow, A. H. (1943). A theory of human motivation. *Psychological Review*, *50*, 370–396. doi: 10.1037/h0054346.

Masten, A. S. (2014). *Ordinary magic: Resilience in development*. New York: The Guilford Press.

McCrea, K. T., & Bulanda, J. J. (2010). Caregiving heuristics: Valuable practitioner knowledge in the context of managing residential care. *Qualitative Social Work*, *9*, 343–363. doi: 10.1177/1473325010367818.

Mehana, M., & Reynolds, A. J. (2004). School mobility and achievement: A meta-analysis. *Children & Youth Services Review*, *26*, 93–119. doi: 10.1016/j.childyouth.2003.11.004.

Meichsner, S. (2021). The ideological underpinnings and political usefulness of residential care for children and young people. *Childhood*, *28*, 459–464. doi: 10.1177/09075682211020069.

Mesman, J., & Emmen, R. A. G. (2021). Cultural perspectives on parenting. In V. A. Weekes-Shackelford & T. Shackelford (Eds.), *The Oxford handbook of evolutionary psychology and parenting* (pp. 97–114). New York: Oxford University Press.

Moore, T., McArthur, M., Death, J., Tilbury, C., & Roche, S. (2017). Young people's views on safety and preventing abuse and harm in residential care: "It's got to be better than home." *Children and Youth Services Review*, *81*, 212–219. doi:10.1016/j.childyouth.2017.08.010

Mota, C. P., & Matos, P. M. (2015). Does sibling relationship matter to self-concept and resilience in adolescents under residential care? *Children and Youth Services Review*, *56*, 97–106. doi: 10.1016/j.childyouth.2015.06.017.

Neagu, M. (2021). *Voices from the silent cradles: Life histories of Romania's looked after children*. Bristol: Policy Press.

Nelson, T. D., Van Dyck, T. R., Lundahl, A., Huefner, J., Thompson, R. W., & Epstein, M. H. (2013). Patterns and correlates of adolescent weight change in residential care. *Children and Youth Services Review*, *35*, 960–965. doi: 10.1016/j.childyouth.2013.03.007.

Nijhof, K. S., Veerman, J. W., Engels, R. C. M. E., & Scholte, R. H. J. (2011). Compulsory residential care: An examination of treatment improvement of individual and family functioning. *Children and Youth Services Review*, *33*, 1779–1785. doi: 10.1016/j.childyouth.2011.05.001.

Nuñez, M., Beal, S. J., & Jacquez, F. (2022). Resilience factors in youth transitioning out of foster care: A systematic review. *Psychological Trauma, 14*(S1), S72–S81. doi: 10.1037/tra0001096

Olsen, R. F., & de Montgomery, C. J. (2018). Revisiting out-of-home placed children's poor educational outcomes—Is school change part of the explanation? *Children and Youth Services Review*, *88*, 103–113. doi: 10.1016/j.childyouth.2018.03.005.

Osei, G. K., & Gorey, K. M. (2019). Peer influences moderated by group home size: Retrospective cohort of youths in Ontario group home care, 2012 to 2016. *Children and Youth Services Review*, *107*, 104564. doi: 10.1016/j.childyouth.2019.104564.

Palareti, L., & Berti, C. (2009). Different ecological perspectives for evaluating residential care outcomes: Which window for the black box? *Children and Youth Services Review*, *31*, 1080–1085. doi: 10.1016/j.childyouth.2009.07.011.

Proeschold-Bell, R. J., Molokwu, N. J., Keyes, C. L. M., Sohail, M. M., Eagle, D. E., Parnell, H., ... Whetten, K. (2019). Caring and thriving: An international qualitative study of caregivers of orphaned and vulnerable children and strategies to sustain positive mental health. *Children and Youth Services Review*, *98*, 143–153. doi: 10.1016/j.childyouth.2018.12.024.

Racine, N., Eirich, R., & Madigan, S. (2022). Fostering resilience in children who have been maltreated: A review and call for translational research. *Canadian Psychology/Psychologie Canadienne*, *63*, 203–213. https://doi.org/10.1037/cap0000312.

Rauktis, M. E., Fusco, R. A., Cahalane, H., Bennett, I. K., & Reinhart, S. M. (2011). "Try to make it seem like we're regular kids": Youth perceptions of restrictiveness in out-of-home care. *Children and Youth Services Review*, *33*, 1224–1233. doi: 10.1016/j.childyouth.2011.02.012.

Refaeli, T., Benbenishty, R., & Eliel-Gev, M. (2013). Youth aging out of residential care in Israel: Readiness for independent living and need for help. *Children and Youth Services Review*, *35*, 1601–1607. doi: 10.1016/j.childyouth.2013.06.014.

Reznikovski-Kuras, A., & Gerasimenko, A. (2020). Identifying best-practice strategies for managing residential caregivers working with children at risk. *International Journal of Child, Youth and Family Studies*, *11*, 96–114. doi: 10.18357/ijcyfs114.2202019990.

Ringle, J. L., Ingram, S. D., & Thompson, R. W. (2010). The association between length of stay in residential care and educational achievement: Results from 5- and 16-year follow-up studies. *Children and Youth Services Review*, *32*, 974–980. doi: 10.1016/j.childyouth.2010.03.022.

Robinson, L. R., Boris, N. W., Heller, S. S., Rice, J., Zeanah, C. H., Clark, C., & Hawkins, S. (2012). The good enough home?: Home environment and outcomes of young maltreated children. *Child & Youth Care Forum*, *41*, 73–88. doi: 10.1007/s10566-011-9157-3.

Robst, J., Rohrer, L., Dollard, N., & Armstrong, M. (2014). Family involvement in treatment among youth in residential facilities: Association with discharge to family-like setting and follow-up treatment. *Journal of Emotional and Behavioral Disorders*, *22*, 190–196. doi: 10.1177/1063426614523651.

Roca, J. S., Garcia, M. J., Biarnés, A. V., & Rodriguez, M. (2009). Analysis of factors involved in the social inclusion process of young people fostered in residential care institutions. *Children and Youth Services Review*, *31*, 1251–1257. doi: 10.1016/j.childyouth.2009.05.010.

Roy, C., Morizot, J., Lamothe, J., & Geoffrion, S. (2020). The influence of residential workers social climate on the use of restraint and seclusion: A longitudinal study in a residential treatment center for youth. *Children and Youth Services Review*, *114*, 105035. doi: 10.1016/j.childyouth.2020.105035.

Sackett, D. L., & Rosenberg, W. M. (1995). On the need for evidence-based medicine. *Journal of the Royal Society of Medicine*, *88*, 620–624. doi: 10.1177/014107689508801105.

Slaatto, A., Kleppe, L. C., Mellblom, A., & Baugerud, G. A. (2023). Youth in residential facilities: "Am I safe?," "Do I matter?," and "Do you care?". *Residential Treatment for Children & Youth*, *40*, 87–108. doi: 10.1080/0886571X.2022.2082628.

Sameroff, A. J., & Rosenblum, K. L. (2006). Psychosocial constraints on the development of resilience. In B. M. Lester, A. Masten, & B. McEwen (Eds.), *Resilience in children. Annals of the New York Academy of Sciences, 1094* (pp. 116–124). Hoboken, NJ: Blackwell. doi: 10.1196/annals.1376.010.

Sekol, I. (2013). Peer violence in adolescent residential care: A qualitative examination of contextual and peer factors. *Children and Youth Services Review*, *35*, 1901–1912. doi: 10.1016/j.childyouth.2013.09.006.

Smith, M. (2009). *Rethinking residential care: Positive perspectives*. Bristol: The Policy Press.

Strijbosch, E. L. L., Van der Helm, G. H. P., van Brandenburg, M. E. T., Mecking, M., Wissink, I. B., & Stams, G. J. J. M. (2014). Children in residential care: Development and validation of a group climate instrument. *Research on Social Work Practice*, *24*, 462–469. doi: 10.1177/1049731513510045.

Sulimani-Aidan, Y. (2018). Present, protective, and promotive: Mentors' roles in the lives of young adults in residential care. *American Journal of Orthopsychiatry*, *88*, 69–77. doi:10.1037/ort0000235

Sulimani-Aidan, Y., & Benbenishty, R. (2011). Future expectations of adolescents in residential care in Israel. *Children and Youth Services Review*, *33*, 1134–1141. doi: 0.1016/j.childyouth.2011.02.006.

Thompson, R. W., Smith, G. L., Osgood, D. W., Dowd, T. P., Friman, G.L., & Daly, D. L. (1996). Residential care: A study of short- long-term educational effects. *Children and Youth Services Review*, *18*, 221–242. doi:10.1016/0190-7409(96)00002-3

Urban, T. H., Jordan, N., Kisiel, C. L., & Fehrenbach, T. (2019). The association between strengths and post-residential treatment needs of youth in the child welfare system. *Children and Youth Services Review*, *99*, 226–234. doi: 10.1016/j.childyouth.2019.02.013.

Ward, A. (2004). Towards a theory of the everyday: The ordinary and the special in daily living in residential care. *Child & Youth Care Forum*, *33*, 209–225. doi: 10.1023/B:CCAR.0000029686.10310.49.

Yeager, D. S., & Dweck, C. S. (2012). Mindsets that promote resilience: When students believe that personal characteristics can be developed. *Educational Psychologist*, *47*, 302–314. doi: 10.1080/00461520.2012.722805.

Yoon, S., Howell, K., Dillard, R., McCarthy, K. S., Napier, T. R., & Pei, F. (2021). Resilience following child maltreatment: Definitional considerations and developmental variations. *Trauma, Violence, and Abuse*, *22*, 541–559. doi: 10.1177/1524838019869094.

Zeller, M., & Köngeter, S. (2012). Education in residential care and in school: A social-pedagogical perspective on the educational attainment of young women leaving care. *Children and Youth Services Review*, *34*, 1190–1196. doi: 10.1016/j.childyouth.2012.01.047.

7 Working Models of Residential Care in Children's Homes

Quality residential care can, then, be defined. We know enough to provide it if we conclude that it is necessary, and we are willing to pay for it. In this chapter I will describe two models of care that have been put into practice in the United States. I have chosen to focus on these two models for several reasons. First, these two models are based on what I consider sound principles of developmental psychology. Thus, they both reflect my own area of expertise, and I am comfortable in presenting and evaluating them. Second, both have been applied widely enough to demonstrate their usefulness. Although there are no definitive randomized clinical trials comparing the models to no treatment, there is significant pre-post and quasi-experimental evidence for each. The Teaching Family Model is included in James' evaluation of "what works" in Chapter 5. It has been used in a wide variety of settings, including children's homes, detention centers, group homes, psychiatric treatment centers, and schools (Casey et al., 2010). The newer CARE model (Holden, 2009; Holden et al., 2010) has been getting substantial attention recently and I have regular contact with a children's home that has been using it for over five years and had a program consistent with the model's principles for nearly two decades prior. Third, the two models, although each based on sound principles, are different in important ways yet similar in essential practices. They offer alternative ways of thinking about training staff and treating children and youth. Finally, I judge both models to be capable of wide dissemination. The child welfare system needs a set of models that can be easily and widely copied. These two models fit those criteria.

This chapter does not provide operational manuals for the models. I will simply provide brief descriptions of their historical and conceptual roots, the essential principles of the models, a representative sample of the literature on their application and effectiveness, and an evaluation of the strengths and weaknesses of each model as it has been used. James, Thompson, and Ringle's (2017) survey of residential care providers shows that while providers were using practices for dealing with individual children and youth and particular program issues, fewer respondents were using milieu-based models like those reviewed in James (2011). Models such as the Teaching Family Model and CARE require extensive staff training, committed

DOI: 10.4324/9781003435709-7

leadership, and careful evaluation. Perhaps attention to these two models will lead more providers to commit to approaches that are supported by research evidence.

The Teaching Family Model

No approach to residential care has received more research attention than the Teaching Family Model. Its features support the reality of high-quality residential care.

Theoretical foundations. The roots of the Teaching Family Model are in behaviorist psychology, specifically, the branch of behaviorism championed by B. F. Skinner (1969), operant conditioning. By the 1960s, Skinnerian behaviorism dominated certain psychology and psychology-related departments in universities. One university where operant conditioning was dominant was the University of Washington. There, a group of psychologists, including Montrose Wolf, began to apply the concepts of operant conditioning from laboratory research with animals to real-life human problems. After a stint on the faculty at Arizona State where he had obtained his PhD, Wolf joined several other behaviorists at the new Department of Human Development at the University of Kansas. By that time, Wolf, with his colleagues, was inventing what became known as "applied behavior analysis" (ABA; Todd & Morris, 1995). ABA researchers developed their own methodology focused on solving practical problems with rigorous observational techniques and single-subject research designs. Wolf was instrumental in developing central tenets of ABA that recognize the power of reinforcers to shape behavior, including attention from others. Among those new ideas were "time out from reinforcement" (removing a child from environments where undesired behaviors were being reinforced by factors such as attention), the idea of "catch them being good" (provide reinforcers for desired behaviors rather than punishing inappropriate behaviors, which often unintentionally reinforced undesired behaviors with attention), and "token economies" (motivational systems using systematic rewards in the form of tokens that can be turned in for tangibles or privileges).

Wolf used these and other techniques in his work with delinquent boys as a community-based alternative to juvenile detention, then began to teach them to parents, therapists, counselors, and others for use with their children and youth in their care. By the early 1970s, Wolf and his colleagues had started The Teaching Families Association (https://www.teaching-family.org/), involving thousands of families who have learned to use ABA principles to improve their families' lives. The program was disseminated widely, often in group homes for youth who would otherwise be in juvenile detention centers, but also in children's homes and schools (Pinkelman & Horner, 2019). More important for our purposes, in 1975 (for the history of the Teaching Family approach, see Fixsen & Blasé, 2019; Kirigin, 2001), Wolf took the principles of what he now called the Teaching Family Model, to Father Flanagan's Boys Town (Wolf, Kirigin, Fixsen, Blasé, & Braukmann, 1995). Boys Town moved residents from dormitories into small cottages with teaching family-trained parents (Hupp, 1985). The model has evolved and been used in what is now Boys Town/Girls Town in training their residential staff and foster care parents ever since.

Central components of the Teaching Family Model. The central components of the model include the use of token economies, self-government systems, a skill teaching style, establishment of mutually reinforcing relationships, and effective administration.

A **token economy** is a teaching tool that uses systematic reinforcement for targeted behaviors. Wolf and his colleagues had had success changing behavior with token economies with a variety of populations, including preschoolers, children and adults with developmental disabilities, psychiatric patients, and others. The economies, based on points, are individualized in terms of the targeted behaviors and the rewards points can be exchanged for objects or privileges. Typical targeted behaviors are following instructions, using appropriate language, completion of chores, and finishing homework. Early research on token economies indicated that they were susceptible to many of the same characteristics as real economies, including inflation. So, in the Teaching Family Model, the use of token economies is faded out for an individual once target behaviors are learned and come under the control of naturally occurring reinforcers.

Wolf and his colleagues were concerned that an "us versus them" culture could develop in cottages between adults and residents. To avoid this, youth are given responsibility for **self-government**, to set their own regulations in daily "family conferences," 30 to 60 minutes in length. There residents learn to set and change rules and define violations and consequences. Peers are given the power to give and take away tokens or points in the token economies. A role in self-governance has proved to be a major correlate of resident satisfaction in research on the Teaching Family Model.

The Teaching Family Model relies on staff members who have learned to interact with residents in a particular **skill teaching style**. The idea of a "style" of relating is not Skinnerian, but in the Teaching Family Model it ensures that there is consistency in how staff relate to residents and provides a positive atmosphere for the rest of the system components. The elements of relationship style include expressions of affection and praise, clear verbal descriptions of, and rationales for, appropriate and inappropriate behaviors and their consequences. Clear feedback, including use of praise, rewards and correction are also important factors in the relationship style. Using this style provides important information to residents. Teacher-parents communicate that they care, that they know about the resident's behavior, and that they will give residents reasons for expectations and performance (consistent with what Baumrind, 2013, calls the "authoritative" style of parenting).

Like "style," the concept of **developing of mutually reinforcing relationships** is a bit soft for a behaviorist. Wolf and his colleagues sought to operationalize the teacher-parent-resident relationship in terms of behavior and reinforcement. For the philosophy of behaviorism, reinforcers are central. To be effective, they must (by circular definition) have value. In the residential care setting, reinforcers get much of their value from the teacher-parent-resident relationship. The "style" elements above enhance reinforcement value through positive associations. The emphasis in interactions is on praise and constructive feedback. If there is a single "law" of effective residential care, it is that outcomes and satisfaction are always related to the strength of the resident-caregiver relationship.

Extensive training of staff members in effective administration is central to the implementation of the Teaching Family Model (Fixsen & Blasé, 2019). Teaching parents are considered professionals and must attain a professional level of expertise. Full implementation of the Teaching Family Model in an organization requires three to five years, usually closer to five.

Research on the Teaching Family Model: Does it work? More than a hundred journal articles have been published on the Teaching Family Model, going back some 50 years. I will focus on some of the more recent work (Daly & Thompson, 2023). There has been no randomized clinical trial with equivalent groups that either received the Teaching Family Model treatment or did not. However, because the Teaching Family Model has been used with so many different residential populations and in so many different settings, residential and non-residential, it is less difficult to make definitive conclusions about it from the quasi-experimental studies available. In some studies, Teaching Family Model homes on the main Boys Town campus or other campuses have been compared to group homes in the community. Farmer, Wagner, Burns, and Murray (2016) found that campus-based homes tend to serve a child welfare population whereas community-based group homes are more likely to serve a psychiatric population. Moreover, the nature of the applied behavior analysis approach is to obtain very specific behavioral data on what individual children and youth are doing, and to chart those data to see if interventions are working. That approach makes it less likely, and perhaps less important, to evaluate programs in more traditional ways.

Because its early applications were often funded with federal grants (a rarity in residential care research), the Teaching Family Model has been subject to internal and external evaluations. Studies from the 1970s and 1980s, mostly using pre-post designs, sometimes with follow-up over short periods, by insiders and outsiders, generally supported the effectiveness of the Teaching Family Model while youth were in residence (see Fixsen & Blasé, 2019; Kingsley, 2006; Kirigin, 2001; Wolf et al., 1995). There were questions early on about its generality beyond the residence period (Braukmann & Wolf, 1987) but more sophisticated statistical analyses ultimately showed that Teaching Family Model residents had lower recidivism rates even in the early studies (Kingsley, 2006). More recently, the evidence has come from varied sources. Simple pre-post group studies (e.g., Larzelere, Daly, Davis, Chmelka, & Handwerk, 2004) show improvement in problem behaviors (both internalizing and externalizing behaviors) while residents are in Teaching Model homes. A meta-analysis of studies with juvenile offenders reveals the Teaching Family Model to be one of just two interventions that are effective (Lipsey & Wilson, 1998). Casey et al. (2010) found that youth transitioning from Boys Town self-reported, compared to norms, average to above average scores on measures of educational/employment skills, self-determination, social support, life skills and hopefulness (however, teachers rated them lower on self-determination).

Some of the firmest support for the Teaching Family Model comes from studies of the educational success of former Boys/Girls Town residents mentioned in Chapter 5. On measures like grades, years of education completed, and attitudes toward education, former residents outperformed those who had been admitted to Boys Town but had not attended (Ringle, Ingram, & Thompson, 2010; Thompson et al., 1996). In addition, studies found that length of stay in residence is positively correlated with continued educational progress. The longer the youth had been in residence, the more likely they were able to successfully continue their educations, including graduating from high school.

Two of the strongest studies of the Teaching Family Model used creative quasi-experimental designs. Lee and Thompson (2008) compared residents from Girls and Boys Town to those who had been in treatment foster care, using a technique called propensity matching. As discussed earlier, a pervasive weakness in research on residential care is the absence of randomized clinical trials that can establish causality between treatments (residential interventions) and outcomes. There are no ethical ways to ensure equivalence between experimental and comparison groups by randomly assigning individuals to groups prior to residency. The propensity matching technique attempts to make group equivalence as likely as possible by matching groups on as many background variables. While lacking the magical equivalence power of random assignment, with large groups, propensity matching gives some confidence that groups are alike before an intervention. Lee and Thompson used 18 background variables (e.g., histories of neglect and abuse, number of prior placements, family characteristics, and demographics). Results show that residents of Girls and Boys Town were more likely to have been favorably discharged, more likely to return to their home, and less likely to experience another placement in the first six months after they were discharged. However, at the six-month follow-up, the groups did not differ in terms of legal involvement or likelihood of being in a home environment (both groups were low on the former).

Farmer, Seifert, Wagner, Burns, and Murray (2017) recognized that while there is considerable evidence that the Teaching Family Model works while youth are in residence, little was known about what happened after they left. They used a variety of measures, including caregiver observations, interviews, and questionnaires in comparing youth from 24 group homes from seven agencies using the Teaching Family Model with youth from 25 homes from seven agencies using an eclectic set of approaches. Most of the youth in the study (mean age of 14.7 years) had been diagnosed with conduct disorders or ADHD. Both groups showed declines in problem behaviors while they were in residence, supporting the general positive influence of good residential care. Follow-up assessments were made a four months and eight months after discharge. On those assessments, the youth from the Teaching Family Model homes continued to show declines in problem behaviors whereas scores of those from the eclectic programs leveled off. Farmer et al. conclude: (a) extended stays in residential care can lead to continuing improvements; and (b) the use of a systematic, comprehensive residential care model like the Teaching Family Model can lead to long-term positive effects.

Overall assessment of the Teaching Family Model. Most of the criticisms of the Teaching Family Model have fallen into one of three categories: general criticisms of residential care; specific criticisms of behavioristic approaches of working with children; and concerns about operational features of the Teaching Family Model and its dissemination.

As we have seen throughout this book, there are those who reject residential care as a means of dealing with any population of children or youth. Among the concerns are that residential care provides an unstimulating environment, that it does not allow caregiver-child attachments or relationships to form, that it is ineffective in changing resident behavior, and that it ignores the individuality of the residents. The charge of ineffectiveness does not stand up well as we saw in Chapter 5 and in the section on research specific to the Teaching Family Model above (also, see Kingsley, 2006). Teaching Family Model advocates point toward the centrality of building the teaching parent-resident relationship in their approach (as pointed out by Wolf et al., 1995, early failures to replicate the Teaching Family Model were due to a failure to establish relationships). The heart of an applied behavior analysis intervention is the development of individualized plans, both in terms of targeted behaviors and selection of reinforcers. The caregiver-resident ratios (typically two caregivers for six to ten residents) and behavioral programming needed in the Teaching Family homes mean that residents are clearly stimulated. A common criticism of residential programs that serve troubled children and youth is negative peer contagion, the idea that peers reinforce inappropriate behavior while there are no models for appropriate behavior (the iatrogenic effect). We dealt with this issue in Chapter 4. Although there is no question that peers sometimes reinforce negative behaviors in unstructured environments, there is little evidence that they do so in structured environments (Huefner, Smith, & Stevens, 2018; Larzelere et al., 2004; Weiss et al., 2005). There is also significant evidence that peers can provide supports for positive behaviors that compete with negative behaviors (Ainsworth & Bath, 2023; Barry & Wentzel, 2006; Huefner et al., 2018; Laursen & Veenstra, 2023).

Applications of behaviorism have always been controversial. It is not surprising that with its use of core operant conditioning principles, that the Teaching Family Model is the target of like criticisms. General philosophical objections to behavioral control are not uncommon, often focusing on reactance responses to attempts at control (e.g., Vander Ven, 2009) or that behaviorist approaches sacrifice dealing with underlying problems to manage behavior (Sinclair, 2005). Specific concerns about the use of token economies (also known as point leveling) include: behavioral approaches can cause alienation and distortion in relationships, including resistance from residents; generalization of the rewarded behaviors does not always occur; programs are inflexible and not individualized, have a punitive tone, can trigger traumatic memories; and they undermine social development by housing troubled peers together (Boldt, Witzel, Russell, & Jones, 2007; Drumm et al., 2013; Rauktis, 2016). Peterson and Huefner (2023), two investigators from Boys Town, respond directly to these concerns. They argue that development of relationships is central to the Teaching Family Model, client resistance is attenuated in the Teaching Family Model because residents are involved in self-government, positive responses from caregivers greatly outnumber negative responses, target behaviors and reward selection are individualized, and generalization is enhanced by fading out of the token economies as youth skills develop and natural reinforcers take over. They also point out that there is no empirical evidence that the Teaching Family Model retraumatizes youth or leads to peer modeling of negative behavior (Huefner et al., 2018). In short, while some individuals do not like behavioral approaches, there is little empirical support for most of their concerns. From early in its history, the creators of the Teaching Family Model moved beyond mechanistic versions of behaviorism. They found that relationships and contexts were essential to success.

It is not easy to start a Teaching Family Model program. As indicated above, it takes three to five years to establish a teaching family home with the appropriate procedures for delivering and monitoring. However, most high-quality residential care requires similar efforts, including the CARE model described next. The resources of the Teaching Family Association help. And the model had been replicated nearly 800 times as of 2007 (Fixsen, Blasé, Timbers, & Wolf, 2007).

Finally, all residential care is criticized for being expensive. The high cost is given as a reason for eliminating residential care (Font & Gershoff, 2020). In response, Huefner et al. (2018) provide an analysis of the long-term cost benefits of the Teaching Family Model that takes into consideration the long-term costs of under-education and under-employment as it relates to length of stay in residential care. Using data from residents who were at Boys Town less than six months versus more than six months, they estimate the return on investment to be $0.36 on the dollar for the short stayers and $3.61 for the long stayers.

The Children and Residential Experiences (CARE) Model

The second model of high-quality residential care I focus on is CARE (Holden, Sellers, & Smith, 2023). It is a product of the Residential Child Care Project of the Bronfenbrenner Center for Translational Research at Cornell University.

The CARE model helps childcare agencies to rethink what they do, at all levels of the organization, based on caregiver-child relationships and developmental principles. CARE is consistent with the argument that the critical component of any intervention with youth is the building of developmental relationships (Bronfenbrenner & Evans, 2000). As Li and Julian (2012) say: "...developmental relationships constitute the active ingredient of effective interventions serving at-risk children and youth across settings...it is time to make developmental relationship the very outcome that is measurable and worth paying for" (pp. 157/164). The question for residential care is whether residential care strengthens or weakens developmental relationships (Costa, Melim, Tagliabue, Mota, & Matos, 2020). The CARE model intervenes at the organizational level, not directly with children or youth (see Anglin, 2011 for a history of the early development of the CARE model).

Theoretical foundations of CARE. The theoretical roots of CARE are in the attachment theory of Ainsworth and Bowlby and their colleagues, the bioecological theory of Bronfenbrenner, the cognitive developmental theory of Vygotsky, and Anglin's thinking about pain and trauma. The most succinct presentation of CARE's approach is found in Holden's (2009) *Children and residential experiences: Creating conditions for change*, the most recent, thoroughly revised, edition of which will be issued in 2023.

At one time, the full name of **attachment theory** was ethological-organizational attachment theory (Waters, 1981). The ethological aspect of the theory reflects the evolutionary importance of attachments. Secure attachments help individuals survive to pass on their genes. Moreover, in some ways, children are "built" to send off signals when in distress and caregivers are "built" to respond to those signals. Attachment is so important that everyone becomes attached to one or more caregiver. What varies is not whether one is attached, but the quality of the attachment. The organizational aspect of the theory reflects the interaction of the attachment system with other systems, including the fear-wariness system, the caregiving system, the peer/social system, and the exploration system, that determine what an individual does in any situation. Attachment theory was originally developed to help understand infant development, but over the past 60 years has become a lifespan theory of development. This is not the place for a full explication of the theory, but a brief review of four basic components will be useful for understanding the CARE model: formation of attachments, internal working models, the interaction of systems, and individual differences. The original versions of attachment theory can be found in Bowlby (1969) and Ainsworth's early summary (Ainsworth, Blehar, Waters, & Wall, 1978). A good source on the development of the theory, especially its applications to post-infant development can be found in the various versions of the *Handbook of Attachment*, especially the most recent edition (Cassidy & Shaver, 2016).

The **formation of attachments** is a fundamental developmental task. Attachment is sometimes confused with imprinting, the phenomenon in nonhuman animals describing how infant animals instinctively bond with caregivers. Human attachments take time to form. Over the first four to six months of life, the infant sends off signals to caregivers (e.g., cries, coos, glances, touches) indicating her needs. If the caregiver consistently picks up the child's signals and responds in a sensitive way (giving the child what they need, not necessarily what they want), the system is working. The child begins to expect that when distressed, there will be an appropriate response. The caregiver provides a safe haven that the child can count on—a secure attachment. Over time, children build up mental representations of their attachments. They use these "internal working models" to set up expectations for interacting with caregivers and peers. These internal models can change over time, but initial models set up expectancies that can influence how they interpret all other relationships (one of the best explanations of the idea of the internal working model can be found in Posada and Waters, 2018).

Developing attachments is not the child's only concern. They also need to find out about their physical environments through exploration and about the people through developing relationships. The child also needs to be wary of potentially harmful threats in the environment. The attachment, exploration, social, and fear/wariness **systems interact** in complex ways. When the fear/wariness system is activated, so is the attachment system, but the exploration and social systems are inhibited. When the exploration or social system is activated, the attachment system is relatively deactivated. There are **individual differences** in how the systems interact with each other that reflect different working models of attachment. When caregivers have consistently responded to the child's needs, the child develops an expectancy that they have a safe haven and can explore their physical and social environments without fear, knowing that the attachment figure will be available if needed. This kind of relationship is a secure attachment. When a caregiver has responded inconsistently or inappropriately to the child's signals, ignored the child or was intrusive, the attachment formed is insecure.

Ainsworth and her colleagues (1978) developed the "Strange Situation" to assess how the various systems interacted in individual infants and toddlers. The general categories identified have since been extended and adapted for older children and adults using various measurement devices. The optimal form of attachment is secure. Insecure forms of attachments include: (a) avoidant attachments, characterized by relationships with the adult and child often do not read each other's signals correctly so that the child may be too independent, unsure in exploration, and generally unconfident; (b) resistant or ambivalent attachments, characterized by child behaviors that are simultaneously demanding contact and pushing the caregiver away, reflecting an uncoordinated set of systems; and (c) disorganized attachments, mixing the other versions of insecurity; the caregivers in disorganized relationships often have been victims of trauma or abuse themselves. Children who have developed secure attachments with at least one caregiver show the best skills in problem solving, developing social relationships with adults and peers, the most positive self-perceptions, and the strongest ability to deal with stress. Many children in the welfare system have histories without secure attachments in the families where they have resided.

The CARE model is used in residential settings for older children and youth, not infants. However, the applications of attachment theory to older children and adults (Cassidy & Shaver, 2016) generally follow the same sorts of internal working models developed in the infant models. The complexities in attachment for children and youth revolve around the dysfunctional insecure attachments and working models of relationships they have often formed throughout their childhoods, particularly when they have been in multiple foster care placements.

Bronfenbrenner's ecological theory was used in Chapter 6 as a framework for thinking about quality environments. His later **bioecological theory** (Bronfenbrenner & Evans, 2000) is closely related to the CARE model principles and to the other theories that have influenced it. This version of the theory has three core propositions. The first is that development is driven by proximal processes (including attachments) that occur through progressively more complex interactions between active individuals and the people, objects, and symbols in their environments. Those processes can result in either competence, the adaptive ability to conduct and control behavior, or dysfunction. Bronfenbrenner calls proximal processes the "engines of development." A corollary of the first proposition is that the outcomes of proximal processes depend on the degree of exposure an individual has to the reciprocal interactions, an echo of attachment theory. Exposure includes how long and how often the exposure occurs, the timing and intensity of the interactions, and whether the interactions are interrupted.

The second proposition of the bioecological theory is that developmental outcomes are a function of the characteristics of the individual, the environmental context, and the environmental changes that occur over time. Finally, the third proposition is that optimal development depends not only on a progressively more complex and challenging set of reciprocal interactions, but on relationships with attachment figures committed to mutual wellbeing.

For Lev **Vygotsky**, a Belarusian psychologist active in the USSR in the 1920s and 1930s, all aspects of the child's development are influenced by the environment the child lives in. A child's thinking is influenced by his or her culture as the representatives of that culture (parents, teachers, older children) interact with the child. The main mechanism for that interaction, of course, is language. Vygotsky (1978) argues that thinking is essentially internalized language. And because language is both a product of and a mediator of the child's culture, thinking is really internalized culture. Much of Vygotsky's work focused on the development of language and thinking during infancy. However, the part of Vygotsky's theory that influences the CARE model concerns his view of how the environment influences the child's increasingly complex thinking through scaffolding or symbolic mediation. The notion is that a knowledgeable adult or even a developmentally advanced peer helps the child develop cognitively through social support. If a child is struggling with a task, the adult might model a partial form of the solution, give a hint, ask a question, leave a gap for the child to fill in or otherwise lead the child toward a solution without giving away the answer.

According to Vygotsky, each member of the interaction has an agenda (a dynamic, changing one) and during the interaction they must negotiate a shared agenda. The agendas are influenced by where each person's thinking is in relation to the task or problem. In Vygotsky's view the child is not at a particular point in development in relation to the task but is in a zone. This zone ranges from not being able to do the task at all to being able to do it with a lot of help, to being able to do it with hints, to being able to do the task independently. If the expert in the interaction can adjust their agenda to a point close enough to where the child's is, and the child is able to first do the task with help and then do it on her own, Vygotsky would say that the child is in the "zone of proximal development." A child in the zone of proximal development is quite different cognitively from a child who does not know anything about a task. The social situation can reveal that the child knows more, and it can be the agent for the child to grow cognitively to full understanding (Vygotsky believed there was another way to learn, through cognitive mediation or what he called scientific concepts, but that need not concern us here). In the CARE model, competence, one of the basic principles, is gained when the careworker (the term used in the CARE model for agency caregivers providing direct care and therapy) interacts with the residents within each one's zone of proximal development, making meaning together in social interactions that get gradually more complex.

James **Anglin's** theoretical contribution to the CARE model is most clearly explained in *Pain, normality and the struggle for congruence: Reinterpreting residential care for children and youth* (Anglin, 2002). Based on extensive experience in and research on group homes, Anglin argues that the guiding concept in the work of group homes is "congruence in service of the children's best interests." The struggle to maintain this congruence involves three interacting dimensions.

The three **basic psychosocial processes** in service of congruence are: (a) creating an extra-familial living environment; (b) responding to residents' pain and pain-based behaviors (both internalizing and externalizing behaviors); and (c) providing a sense of normality.

The psychosocial processes interact with **11 interactional dynamics**. These dynamics are the key ingredients for the caregiver-resident relationship. They are: (a) listening and responding with respect; (b) communicating a framework for understanding; (c) building rapport and relationship; (d) establishing structure, routine, and expectations; (e) inspiring commitment; (f) offering emotional and developmental support; (g) challenging thinking and action;

(h) sharing power and decision-making; (i) respecting personal space and time; (j) discovering and uncovering potential; and (k) providing resources. These dynamics provide specific guidance on how to treat residents who are dealing with pain. Note their correspondence with the characteristics of quality described in Chapter 6. They also are fundamental to the nature of relationships in the CARE model.

Anglin argues that the processes and dynamics need to work at every **level of a group home operation.** That includes extra-agency activities (interactions with government bodies, boards, etc.); management (the home's administration, human resources, etc.); supervision (those immediately over direct care); careworkers, and the youth and their families in their daily living. Like Bronfenbrenner's theory, this dimension of Anglin's framework indicates the importance of the ecology of residential care.

CARE principles and processes. The CARE model is designed to help caregiving agencies to reorganize at what Anglin would call all levels of group home organization and Bronfenbrenner would call the microsystem to the macrosystem. Using the CARE model means change, reallocating resources, resetting priorities, and creating new organizational cultures whenever necessary. The training is manualized. CARE provides multiple training sessions with an implementation team from the organization and on-site technical assistance and feedback based on observations is available throughout the implementation. Three processes are important to the implementation of CARE (Holden & Sellers, 2019). First, the implementation is characterized by data-informed decisions at all levels. Questionnaires and observations are used with all levels of the organization's staff as well as with residents and their families (when appropriate). Second, reflective practice is encouraged by all participants. Rather than doing things habitually, staff members are encouraged to think about what they are doing and why they are doing it. Third, at all levels, participatory management involves administration, careworkers, and children and youth in decision making.

While the processes are important, the heart of CARE is the use of six basic principles. The assumption is that the implementation of the model will work to the degree that these principles infuse all levels of the organization. Each of these principles is based on one or more of the theories outlined above.

Principle 1, "developmentally focused," is that children and youth of different ages must be treated in accordance with their developmental status. Attachment theory suggests that attachments take qualitatively different forms at different ages. Early on, relationships with caregivers are primary. Later, relationships with peers and adults, such as teachers and coaches, increase in importance. Vygotsky's theory suggests that children and youth perform best within what he called the zone of proximal development. The adults in the resident's life should be challenging the child or youth, consistent with Bronfenbrenner's increasing complex interactions, but not too challenging. As Vygotsky describes, they "scaffold" the child's interactions with the environment by adjusting challenge to the child's ability to handle the challenge, teaching missing skills needed for success. Challenge motivates the individual and is most effective when social supports are available. Adults need to know when it is appropriate to back off and let the child work independently. If adults are intrusive, the child is less likely to be able to work independently.

Principle 2, "family involved," states that whenever possible, residential care needs to facilitate appropriate interactions with family members. In children's homes, the residents are often there because they cannot have direct contact with their immediate families as ordered by a court. However, children's homes are often where sibling groups can be placed. Regular contact with siblings may be an important source of support (Davidson-Arad & Klein, 2011), including attachments. There may be extended family who cannot take children or youth in but who can maintain contact, often grandparents. Sometimes residents can have limited, supervised contact with immediate family members. In the CARE model, it is important that careworkers monitor possible consequences of that contact.

Principle 3, "relationship based," is based on attachment theory and Anglin's framework, both of which support the centrality of the relationships residents form when in care. Bronfenbrenner's proposition about long-term reciprocal commitments also supports this principle. Many of the children and youth in residential care have formed insecure attachments in their families of origin. Many residents of children's homes have faced multiple placements where secure attachments were not made. Careworkers may find it difficult to establish relationships with those whose working models of relationship do not include the sensitive reading of signals and reciprocity. A secure base/safe haven can be provided if careworkers make themselves readily available, invest time and emotional resources in residents, and treat them with respect (Feeney & Collins, 2015; Izzo et al., 2014). It is important that residential care agencies ensure stability of care so trust can be built over time.

Principle 4, "competence centered," is an outcome of the previous two principles. The purpose of being developmentally focused and relationship based is to enhance the social and cognitive competence of residents. Many residents come to care with checkered educational histories, especially those who have experienced multiple foster placements. Many residents also come into care with volatile social histories. Those with insecure attachments are likely to have poor peer relations. Developmentally appropriate educational strategies and social skills often need to be explicitly taught. High but realistic expectations and opportunities for success in educational, social, and recreational activities begin to build self-competence (Harter, 2012). Experiences that teach self-regulation skills and empathy can lead to self-efficacy and, eventually, self-confidence. In Bronfenbrenner's terms, proximal processes should lead to competence, not dysfunction.

Principle 5, "trauma informed," reflects one of the key influences Anglin has had on the CARE model: the awareness of how much of the behavior and misbehavior of residents in care can be traced to pain. The very fact that a child or youth is in care suggests a history of trauma. Abuse, neglect, loss of parents, trouble with the law, and other causes of pain need to be understood and addressed. Therapy is frequently required. Environments must be modified to reduce stress and avoid triggers to residents' sources of pain. Loss, physical, social, and emotional needs to be acknowledged by the residents and those who care for them. The sources of residents' pain need to be sought less in the child than in what has happened to them. Regularly exercising Anglin's interactional dynamics helps careworkers to aid in the expression and management of pain. The aim of CARE is to help staff members to help residents build resiliency. In the CARE model, it also is important that direct care providers have opportunities to deal with the pain they experience themselves from working with those experiencing pain (Modlin, 2019).

Finally, **Principle 6, "ecologically oriented,"** based on both Bronfenbrenner's ecological theory and Anglin's perspective, stresses that children and youth are influenced by all layers of their environments. CARE principles apply to all aspects of an organization. A basic assumption is that a resident's progress will reflect what is happening in their immediate environments (microsystems) but also at the various levels of the organization in charge of their care. A carefully tended physical environment and intelligent use of space can help normalize the resident's experience. Residents should have ownership in their room and common rooms, choices in room decorations, and in clothing. Rich recreational opportunities enhance, physical, social, and emotional development through opportunities for challenge, success, and communication. Little things, like celebrating success, birthdays, and holidays help in the building of relationships.

Research on the CARE Model. Theoretically, CARE should work. Does it? There is much less research on the CARE model than what is available for the Teaching Family Model. It is relatively new and all the available research to date has been in-house. One of the first empirical papers from the CARE team focused on a single large therapeutic care residence for children and youth eight to 18 years of age. Nunno, Smith, Martin and Butcher (2015) implemented the CARE model with the staff in the residential, emergency shelter, and day student programs at the residence. The agency had administrative records on the use of physical restraints for six years before and six years after the implementation of CARE. In both the residential and shelter service components, restraint incidents dropped after the CARE implementation and continued to decline until the fifth year when the rate flattened. For the day student component, incidents increased after implementation and did not begin to decline until the third-year post-implementation. The investigators conclude that the results provide credible evidence for the effectiveness of the CARE intervention.

A larger scale study of CARE is reported by Izzo, Smith, Sellers, Holden and Nunno (2016). The researchers studied two cohorts of agencies in a quasi-experimental design. The agencies served mostly residents who had been referred through the child welfare system. All the careworkers worked one- or two-week shifts, full time (thus, they best fit the category of children's homes). Data for five Cohort 1 agencies were collected for 12 months before the CARE implementation and for 36 months afterward. The agencies in Cohort 2 were kept on a wait list for a year, then data were collected in the same pattern. The unit of analysis was agency, not staff or resident. The dependent variables were behavioral incidents, including threats or physical aggression toward staff and toward peers, self-harming acts or threats, property destruction, and incidents of running away. There were significant decreases in all five categories for Cohort 1. For Cohort 2, there were declines after CARE implementation in incidents of aggression toward staff, property destruction, and running away, but not for aggression toward peers or self-harm.

The Nunno et al. and Izzo et al. studies show declines in negative behaviors after CARE implementation but do not provide evidence about the mechanisms for the change. A key principle in the CARE model is the building of careworker-resident relationships. Izzo, Smith, Sellers, Holden, and Nunno (2020) investigated residents' perceived relationship quality with direct care staff before and after CARE implementation with the 11 agencies that participated in the Izzo et al. (2016) study and two additional sites, one in each cohort. Children completed two questionnaires that tapped their perceptions of their careworkers' sensitivity to the child's needs, emotional availability, responsiveness, autonomy support, growth promotion, punitive attitudes, and other indicators of attachment and relationship quality. The researchers also tested the role of child demographic and organizational climate moderators. The perceived quality of child-adult relationship increased each year after CARE implementation. A particularly interesting finding is that the only significant moderator was the number of previous child placements. Those residents who had experienced the most placements showed the largest increases in perceived relationship quality of daily interactions with direct care workers.

The staff data from the study reported in Izzo et al. (2020) are reported by Izzo, Smith, Sellers, Holden and Nunno (2022). The implicit theories staff members have about child development and childcare influence how they interpret and respond to resident behavior. The investigators assessed staff knowledge of the CARE model, their endorsement of beliefs about child development and care, and also asked children to report on a questionnaire about how well staff practices reflected a relational approach. Across years and agencies, staff members showed more knowledge of CARE, were more likely to endorse behaviors consistent with a relational approach and were less likely to endorse behaviors that would interfere with a relational approach. Self-reported practices consistent with a relational approach did not show a CARE-related change until the third year.

Overall assessment of CARE. The usefulness of the CARE model will not be apparent to those who reject residential care of any kind. The data base in support of the CARE model is thin but encouraging. All the studies have come from the Cornell group. Only relatively weak quasi-experimental designs have been used. There are no studies involving direct observation of careworker-resident interactions. The model does not make residential care cheaper. On the other hand, CARE has a strong base in fundamental theories of child and youth development. It appears to be readily exportable. It reflects values consistent with those important to those who are drawn to childcare.

The Teaching Family Model and CARE Compared

There are important differences between the two models of residential care presented here. The Teaching Family Model has been much more widely used and researched. The theoretical foundations for the two models represent different ends of many dimensions of psychological theories. The Teaching Family Model comes from the behavioristic, contextual side. CARE is more cognitive and developmental. But they are similar in important ways too. Both see an intimate but professional resident-careworker relationship as the active ingredient of the intervention. Both are ecological in orientation and stress positive interactions with residents. Operationally, both require extensive training of professional careworkers. They are both data-oriented, though in different ways. Both require an agency give a three- to-five-year commitment to be fully operational. Both models put a priority on hearing from residents. Either is a solid choice.

References

Ainsworth, F., & Bath, H. (2023). Therapeutic residential care in Australia: A new dawn or more of the same? In J. K. Whittaker, L. Holmes, J. F. del Valle, & S. James (Eds.), *Revitalizing residential care for children and youth: Cross-national trends and challenges* (pp. 391–404). New York: Oxford University Press. doi: 10.1093/oso/9780197644300.003.0026.

Ainsworth, M. D. S., Blehar, M. C., Waters, E., & Wall, S. (1978). *Patterns of attachment: A psychological study of the strange situation.* Hillsdale, NJ: Erlbaum.

Anglin, J. P. (2002). *Pain, normality, and the struggle for congruence: Reinterpreting residential care for children and youth.* New York: Haworth Press.

Anglin, J. P. (2011). *Translating the Cornell CARE program model into practice: Lessons from the pioneer agencies on changing agency cultures and care practice.* Retrieved from: http://rccp.cornell.edu/_assets/Translating%20the%20CARE%20Program%20Model%20into%20Practice%20James%20Anglin.pdf.

Barry, C. M., & Wentzel, K. R. (2006). Friend influence on prosocial behavior: The role of motivational factors and friendship characteristics. *Developmental Psychology, 42*, 153–163. doi: 10.1037/0012-1649.42.1.153.

Baumrind, D. (2013). Authoritative parenting revisited: History and current status. In R. E. Larzelere, A. S. Morris, & A. W. Harrist (Eds.), *Authoritative parenting: Synthesizing nurturance and discipline for optimal child development* (pp. 11–34). Washington, DC: American Psychological Association. doi: 10.1037/13948-002.

Boldt, R. W., Witzel, M., Russell, C., & Jones, V. (2007). Replacing coercive power with relationship power. *Reclaiming Children and Youth, 15*, 243–248. Retrieved from: https://cyc-net.org/cyc-online/cyconline-nov2009-boldt.html.

Bowlby, J. (1969). *Attachment and loss, Volume 1: Attachment.* New York: Basic Books.

Braukmann, C. J., & Wolf, M. M. (1987). Behaviorally based group homes for juvenile offenders. In E. K. Morris & C. J. Braukmann (Eds.), *Behavioral approaches to crime and delinquency: A handbook of application, research, and concepts* (pp. 135–159). New York: Plenum.

Bronfenbrenner, U., & Evans, G. W. (2000). Developmental science in the 21st century: Emerging questions, theoretical models, research designs and empirical findings. *Social Development*, *9*, 115–125. doi: 10.1111/1467-9507.00114.

Casey, K. J., Reid, R., Trout, A. L., Duppong Hurley, K., Chmelka, M. B., & Thompson, R. (2010). The transition status of youth departing residential care. *Child & Youth Care Forum*, *39*, 323–340. doi: 10.1007/s10566-010-9106-6.

Cassidy, J., & Shaver, P. R. (2016). *Handbook of attachment: Theory, research, and clinical applications* (3rd ed.). New York: Guilford Press.

Costa, M., Melim, B., Tagliabue, S., Mota, C. P., & Matos, P. M. (2020). Predictors of the quality of the relationship with caregivers in residential care. *Children and Youth Services Review*, *108*, 104579. doi: 10.1016/j.childyouth.2019.104579.

Daly, D. L., & Thompson, R. W. (2023). A review of the Teaching Family Model/Boys Town Family Home Program. In J. K. Whittaker, L. Holmes, J. F. del Valle, & S. James (Eds.), *Revitalizing residential care for children and youth: Cross-national trends and challenges* (pp. 154–167). New York: Oxford University Press. doi: 10.1093/oso/9780197644300.003.0011.

Davidson-Arad, B., & Klein, A. (2011). Comparative well being of Israeli youngsters in residential care with and without siblings. *Children and Youth Services Review*, *33*, 2152–2159. doi: 10.1016/j.childyouth.2011.06.022.

Drumm, R. D., Coombs, R. S., Hargrove, T. D., Crumley, L. P., Cooper, L., & Foster, T. (2013). "You leave in a body bag or you leave on the points system": Participant perceptions of a points and levels system of behavior management. *Residential Treatment for Children & Youth*, *30*, 262–279. doi: 10.1080/0886571X.2013.842028.

Farmer, E. M. Z., Seifert, H., Wagner, H. R., Burns, B. J., & Murray, M. (2017). Does model matter?: Examining change across time for youth in group homes. *Journal of Emotional and Behavioral Disorders*, *25*, 119–128. doi: 10.1177/1063426616630520.

Farmer, E. M. Z., Wagner, H. R., Burns, B. J., & Murray, M. (2016). Who goes where?: Exploring factors related to placement among group homes. *Journal of Emotional and Behavioral Disorders*, *24*, 54–63. doi: 10.1177/1063426615585082.

Feeney, B. C., & Collins, N. L. (2015). A new look at social support: A theoretical perspective on thriving through relationships. *Personality and Social Psychology Review*, *19*, 113–147. doi: 10.1177/1088868314544222.

Fixsen, D. L., & Blasé, K. A. (2019). The Teaching-Family Model: The first 50 years. *Perspectives on Behavioral Science*, *42*, 189–211. doi: 10.1007/s40614-018-0168-3.

Fixsen, D. L., Blasé, K. A., Timbers, G. D., & Wolf, M. M. (2007). In search of program implementation: 792 replications of the Teaching-Family Model. *The Behavior Analyst Today*, *8*, 96–110. doi: 10.1037/h0100104.

Font, S. A., & Gershoff, E. (2020). Foster care: How we can, and should, do more for maltreated children. *SRCD Social Policy Report*, *33*(3). doi: 10.1002/sop2.10.

Harter, S. (2012). *The construction of the self: Developmental and sociocultural foundations* (2nd ed.). New York: Guilford Press.

Holden, M. J. (2009). *Children and residential experiences: Creating conditions for change*. Arlington, VA: Child Welfare League of America.

Holden, M. J., Izzo, C. V., Nunno, M. A., Smith, E. G., Endres, T., Holden, J. C., & Kuhn, F. (2010). Children and residential experiences: A comprehensive strategy for implementing a research-informed program model for residential care. *Child Welfare*, *89*, 131–149. PMID: 20857884.

Holden, M. J., & Sellers, D. E. (2019). An evidence-based program model for facilitating therapeutic responses to pain-based behavior in residential care. *International Journal of Child, Youth and Family Studies*, *10*, 63–80. doi: 10.18357/ijcyfs102-3201918853.

Holden, M. J., Sellers, D. E., & Smith, E. G. (2023). The CARE Program model. In J. K. Whittaker, L. Holmes, J. F. del Valle, & S. James (Eds.), *Revitalizing residential care for children and youth: Cross-national trends and challenges* (pp. 139–153). New York: Oxford University Press. doi: 10.1093/oso/9780197644300.003.0010.

Huefner, J. C., Smith, G. L., & Stevens, A. L. (2018). Positive and negative peer influence in residential care. *Journal of Abnormal Child Psychology*, *46*, 1161–1169. doi: 10.1007/s10802-017-0353-y.

Hupp, R. P. (1985). *The new Boys Town: The story of Father Flanagan's Boys' Home and how its programs were reshaped to meet the complicated and challenging needs of today's troubled youth*. New York: The Newcomen Society of the United States.

Izzo, C. V., Aumand, B. N., Cash, B. M., McCabe, L. A., Holden, M. J., & Bhattacharjee, M. (2014). Exploration of the youth-adult relationship in residential care: Small glimpses from a large sample of youth. *International Journal of Child and Family Welfare*, *15*, 10–23. Retrieve from https://ugp.rug.nl/IJCFW/article/view/37854.

Izzo, C. V., Smith, E. G., Holden, M. J., Norton, C. I., Nunno, M. A., & Sellers, D. E. (2016). Intervening at the setting level to prevent behavioral incidents in residential child care: Efficacy of the CARE program model. *Prevention Science*, *17*, 554–564. doi: 10.1007/s11121-016-0649-0.

Izzo, C. V., Smith, E. G., Sellers, D. E., Holden, M. J., & Nunno, M. A. (2020). Improving relationship quality in group care settings: The impact of implementing the CARE model. *Children and Youth Services Review*, *109*, 104623. doi: 10.1016/j.childyouth.2019.104623.

Izzo, C. V., Smith, E. G., Sellers, D. E., Holden, M. J., & Nunno, M. A. (2022). Promoting a relational approach to residential child care through an organizational program model: Impacts of CARE implementation on staff outcomes. *Children & Youth Services Review*, *132*, 106330. doi: 10.1016/j.childyouth.2021.106330.

James, S. (2011). What works in group care? —A structured review of treatment models for group homes and residential care. *Children and Youth Services Review*, *33*, 308–321. doi: 10.1016/j.childyouth.2010.09.014.

James, S., Thompson, R. W., & Ringle, J. L. (2017). The implementation of evidence-based practices in residential care: Outcomes, processes, and barriers. *Journal of Emotional and Behavioral Disorders*, *25*, 4–18. doi: 10.1177/1063426616687083.

Kingsley, D. (2006). The Teaching-Family Model and post-treatment recidivism: A critical review of the conventional wisdom. *International Journal of Behavioral Consultation and Therapy*, 2, 481–497. doi: 10.1037/h0101002.

Kirigin, K. A. (2001). The Teaching-Family Model: A replicable system of care. *Residential Treatment for Children & Youth*, *18*, 99–111. doi: 10.1300/J007v18n03_09.

Larzelere R. E., Daly, D. L., Davis, J. L., Chmelka, M. B., & Handwerk, M. L. (2004). Outcome evaluation of Girls and Boys Town's Family Home Program. *Education and Treatment of Children*, *27*, 130–149. Retrieved from: https://www.jstor.org/stable/42899792.

Laursen, B., & Veenstra, R. (2023). In defense of peer influence: The unheralded benefits of conformity. *Child Development Perspectives*, *17*, 74–80. doi: 10.1111/cdep.12477.

Lee, B. R., & Thompson, R. (2008). Comparing outcomes for youth in treatment foster care and family-style group care. *Children and Youth Services Review*, *30*, 746–757. doi: 10.1016/j.childyouth.2007.12.002.

Li, J., & Julian, M. M. (2012). Developmental relationships as the active ingredient: A unifying working hypothesis of '"what works"' across intervention settings. *American Journal of Orthopsychiatry*, *82*, 157–166. doi: 10.1111/j.1939-0025.2012.01151.x.

Lipsey, M. W., & Wilson, D. B. (1998). Effective intervention for serious juvenile offenders: A synthesis of research. In R. Loeber & D. P. Farrington (Eds.), *Serious and violent juvenile offenders: Risk factors and successful interventions* (pp. 313–345). Thousand Oaks, CA: Sage.

Modlin, H. (2019). Managing pain in residential care: A developmental analysis. *International Journal of Child, Youth and Family Studies*, *10*, 45–62. doi: 10.18357/ijcyfs102-3201918852.

Nunno, M. A., Smith, E. G., Martin, W. R., & Butcher, S. (2015). Benefits of embedding research into practice: An agency-university collaboration. *Child Welfare*, *94*, 113–133. Retrieved from: https://www.proquest.com/docview/1949558663?pq-origsite=summon.

Peterson, J. C., & Huefner, J. C. (2023). Token economies in residential care systems: Are they bad practice? *Residential Treatment for Children and Youth*, *40*, 261–280. doi: 10.1080/0886571X.2022.2066043.

Pinkelman, S. E., & Horner, R. H. (2019). Applying lessons from the Teaching Family Model: Positive Behavioral Interventions and Supports (PBIS). *Perspectives on Behavioral Science*, *42*, 233–240. doi: 10.1007/s40614-019-00199-x.

Posada, G. E., & Waters, H. S. (2018). The mother-child attachment partnership in early childhood: Secure base behavioral and representational processes: I. Introduction: The co-construction of mother–child attachment relationships in early childhood. *Monographs of the Society for Research in Child Development*, *83*(4), 7–21. doi: 10.1111/mono.12388.

Rauktis, M. E. (2016). "When you first get there, you wear red": Youth perceptions of point and level systems in group home care. *Child & Adolescent Social Work Journal*, *33*, 91–102. doi: 10.1007/s10560-015-0406-4.

Ringle, J. L., Ingram, S. D., & Thompson, R. W. (2010). The association between length of stay in residential care and educational achievement: Results from 5- and 16-year follow-up studies. *Children and Youth Services Review*, *32*, 974–980. doi: 10.1016/j.childyouth.2010.03.022.

Sinclair, I. (2005). Going home or staying away: What is best for long-stay foster children? In N. Axford, V. Berry, M. Little, & L. Morpeth (Eds.), *Forty years of research, policy and practice in children's services: A festschrift for Roger Bullock* (pp. 93–105). Oxford: Wiley.

Skinner, B. F. (1969). *Contingencies of reinforcement: A theoretical analysis*. New York: Appleton-Century-Crofts.

Thompson, R. W., Smith, G. L., Osgood, D. W., Dowd, T. P., Friman, G.L., & Daly, D. L. (1996). Residential care: A study of short- long-term educational effects. *Children and Youth Services Review*, *18*, 221–242. doi: 10.1016/0190-7409(96)00002-3.
Todd, J. T., & Morris, E. K. (Eds.). (1995). *Modern perspectives on B.F. Skinner and contemporary behaviorism*. Westport, CT: Greenwood Press.
Vander Ven, K. (2009). Why focusing on control BACKFIRES: A systems perspective. *Reclaiming Children and Youth*, *17*(4), 8–12. Retrieved from: https://www.proquest.com/docview/214192260?pq-origsite=summon.
Vygotsky, L. S. (1978). *Mind in society: The development of higher psychological processes*. Cambridge, MA: Harvard University Press.
Waters, E. (1981). Traits, behavioral systems, and relationships: Three models of infant mother attachment. In K. Immelmann, G. W. Barlow, L. Petrinovich, & M. Main (Eds.), *Behavioral development / the Bielefeld Interdisciplinary Project* (pp. 621–650). Cambridge: Cambridge University Press. doi: 10.1002/dev.420160311.
Weiss, B., Caron, A., Ball, S., Tapp, J., Johnson, M., & Weisz, J. R. (2005). Iatrogenic effects of group treatment for antisocial youth. *Journal of Consulting and Clinical Psychology*, *73*, 1036–1044.
Wolf, M. M., Kirigin, K. A., Fixsen, D. L., Blasé, K. A., & Braukmann, C. J. (1995). The Teaching-Family Model: A case study in data-based program development and refinement (and dragon wrestling). *Journal of Behavior Management*, *15*, 11–68. doi: 10.1300/J075v15n01_04.

8 A Good Place to Grow

My aim when I started this project was to determine if the strongly negative view of residential care for children whose biological families could not or should not care for them was justified. By justified, I mean whether the research supported the negative view and whether the positive I have witnessed are ephemeral. I was well aware of scandals concerning particular residential programs. I was also aware of scandals involving every other kind of care, including foster care, adoptions, and families of origin. I was not interested in engaging in a war of anecdotes. I have heard many stories, good and bad, from dozens of residents in and after care. While residents need to be heard (and I have included many references in this book to studies where they are), individual testimonies are not enough to condemn or support residential care. My examination of the research literature has been an education for me. Like most education, it has led me to a more complex, nuanced view than I started with. I will sum up what I have learned in eight propositions I think are reasonable.

Conclusions

Proposition 1. The Negative View of Residential Care Is Real

There is a highly negative view of residential care in the academic worlds of social work, law, and clinical psychology and in the worlds of child advocacy agencies and organizations. Yet, one judge in the welfare system who may be more representative than some think (Moriarty, 1999) lamented the lack of residential care as an option in her decisions, saying that the myth of damaging institutionalization pervades the thinking of social workers and the law. There are, just as clearly, specific forms and instantiations of residential care that deserve approbation. An obvious categorical example in the United States and Canada is the boarding schools that were designed to de-culture native children (e.g., Gray & Cote, 2019). There are also many examples of particular group homes and, especially, residences designed for juvenile offenders, that were and are poorly staffed and managed. However, my focus

DOI: 10.4324/9781003435709-8

has been on the published peer-reviewed literature based in empirical research. There you see many introductory statements of a highly defensive nature and reviews that begin with the supposition that all residential care is irrevocably bad. Coming from the Scottish context, Smith (2010) cited Ferguson (2007): "*it is beyond question* that the entire industrial and reformatory regime was an abusive and cruel one" (p. 304, my emphasis). Smith himself pointed out that

> Child care policy over the past 20 years *has been predicated* on assumptions of widespread institutional abuse. These have been used to legitimate a wholesale shift to fostering with resultant multiple placement breakdowns, which has manifestly not protected children from 'institutional' abuse.
>
> (Smith, 2010, p. 314, my emphasis)

As mentioned earlier, Smith notes that Scotland had to close a phone helpline begun to give advice to victims of historical residential abuse when it received only a single call in three months.

The hostility toward residential care in the United States has been clearest in the legislative committee work and lobbying efforts like Richard Wexler's detailed in Chapter 2 and the work of groups like the Annie E. Casey Foundation that led to the passing of the Family First Prevention Services Act. The limitation of federal funding in the United States to only short-term residential care shows unambiguous animus toward residential care. The principle that children and youth should be moved out of residential care as quickly as possible is based on a prejudice that residential care cannot provide a family-like environment, despite what alumni have reported for generations (e.g., McKenzie's work; Neagu, 2021). Without access to high-quality residential care, many children and youth are robbed of the opportunity to develop stable relationships with caring adults, peers, schools, and communities. Failing to discriminate among care environments based on quality helps no child.

The goal of many of those who oppose a role for residential care is the outright elimination of all forms of residential care (see the discussion of Goldman et al., 2020, Chapter 4). That is true even with the availability of research that suggests strongly that residential care is an important component of a complete child welfare system. Discussing the Australian experience of attaining "the dream—no more residential care," Ainsworth and Hansen (2005) note that the dream had "gone disastrously wrong" (p. 197). "Australian experience shows that a mature child care and protection system has to have some residential education and treatment programmes...Foster care, in all its varieties, is not enough" (p. 198). The main concern with residential care may be its cost. Yet, one reason residential care is so expensive is that it has been used as a last resort, as in Australia, reserved for the children with the most difficult backgrounds and greatest needs.

Occasionally there is recognition that the case against residential care is ideologically based, not based on research. For example, Alpert and Meezan (2012) say:

> Child welfare theorists and practice experts in the United States have coalesced around the *philosophical* conclusion that when children cannot remain safely at home they should be placed in family settings whenever possible; congregate care should only be used to deliver time-limited services to children whose special needs require more intensive treatment in a restricted setting (Child Welfare League of America (CWLA), 2005). Federal child welfare policy has embraced this perspective, as well; in 1980, the Adoption Assistance and Child Welfare Act (AACWA) emphasized that children in foster care should be placed in the least restrictive and most family-like environment possible. Though it was largely silent on the specific use of congregate care, AACWA was clear that "[r]esidential care was to be a short-term intervention for troubled children and youth who were on their way to more permanent, family-based settings".
>
> (Alpert & Meezan, 2012, p. 1519, emphasis mine; Courtney & Hughes-Heuring, 2010 (*sic*), p. 182)

Proposition 2. The Negative View of Residential Care of All Types for Children of All Ages Is Based Largely on the Overgeneralization of Research on Infants and Very Young Children Raised in Extreme Environments

The modern hostility toward residential care stems from an overgeneralization of research on infants raised in extremely deprived settings. This is not a close call. The literature on residential care is replete with generalizations across ages, settings, countries, programs, and populations of children and youth, all in problematic ways (Findley, Kikuta, & Denly, 2021; Lucas, 2003). In Chapter 4, we saw how the infant work figured prominently in the Consensus Statement of the Orthopsychiatric Association and the findings of the Lancet Group Commission. The Orthopsychiatric Consensus statement (Dozier et al., 2014) is applied to children of all ages in all types of residential care even though their review hardly touches on practices in the United States, Canada or the United Kingdom or care for older children and youth anywhere. Much of the negative literature about residential care creates a false dichotomy between family and residential care reflecting what Macarov (2008) called a quasi-religious belief that children can only thrive in families. These idealized families are headed by parents who always use just the right amount of warmth, control, and communication whereas residential care is always staffed by unavailable, inflexible, insensitive shift workers. The negative literature also relies too much on limited and challenged research on iatrogenic effects of peers and the Israeli kibbutzim.

The Lancet Group Commission (Goldman et al., 2020) conclusions are bold and stated without conditions. *All* residential care except for small, specialized groups, should eventually close. Like the Ortho consensus statement, it is founded on inappropriately generalized findings. The Commission's statement is based largely on the ungeneralizable results of the Bucharest Early Intervention Project and the equally ungeneralizable van IJzendoorn et al. (2020) meta-analyses. The former generalizes only to similar residential environments for infants and young children. The meta-analyses collapse research, most of it conducted with infants and young children, over 65 years, dozens of countries (little from the United States or Canada, much from Romania, Russia, India, and Turkey) in plainly different but mostly unknown care environments, using varying outcome measures of varying degrees of reliability and validity. The results of the Bucharest Early Intervention Project and van IJzendoorn et al.'s meta-analyses should be generalized with great care and with many conditions. Those cautions are not in the Lancet Group Commission's report.

Other publications make similarly unconditional statements. For example, in an influential monograph from the Society for Research in Child Development (McCall, van IJzendoorn, Juffer, Groark, & Groza, 2011), the editors indicate that "Older children and adolescents in institutions and children residing in institutions in high-resource countries are not covered," (p. 6). Yet a bold, unconditional statement is made just two pages later: "Children exposed to institutional care do not receive the type of nurturing and stimulating environment needed for normal growth and healthy psychological development" (van IJzendoorn et al., 2011, p. 8).

The Sherr, Roberts, and Gandhi (2017) research on child violence experiences (Exhibit 3, Chapter 4) should also not be overgeneralized. It is a given that those in residential care should not experience violence. Perhaps the key feature of Sherr's review is that residential care abuse can be greatly reduced or eliminated with proper staff training. If we adhere to the kind of high-quality care outlined in Chapters 6 and 7, abuse will be extremely rare, surely much rarer than it is in the families from which residents frequently come. Sherr et al.'s focus on violence as neglect or deprivation in the reviews of Johnson and van IJzendoorn reflects many of the issues raised about the Orthopsychiatric Consensus Statement and the Lancet Group Commission papers. The results of the studies covered should not be generalized to most residential care as it has been practiced in the United States, Canada, the United Kingdom, or many other countries in the past 50 years. The facile generalization of findings across populations and settings is in direct contradiction to basic research standards and to the wise calls in developmental psychology for understanding children's lived experience (e.g., Rogoff, Dahl, & Callanan, 2018).

I am not the first to note the overgeneralization problem (see Holmes, Connolly, Mortimer, & Hevesi, 2018, and a sophisticated treatment of the generalization issue in James, 2011). While recognizing the detrimental effects of extreme deprivation, Huynh (2019, p. 100) points out that

> ... these studies of infants in a very specific and negative caregiving environment have often been generalized by policymakers to justify a belief that all residential care settings across countries and continents must have the same poor caregiving characteristics: high child-to-caregiver ratios, shift work, low compensation for caregivers, regimented and non-individualized care, and a lack of psychological investment in the children.

Proposition 3. The Inappropriate Generalization of Findings Has Real Consequences for Children and Youth

The Orthopsychiatric Consensus, the Lancet Group Commission, and the United States' Family First Prevention Services Act make strong statements against residential care with unfortunate consequences. Those consequences can be seen plainly in a policy paper authored by some of the authors of the Ortho statement (Dozier, Zeanah, Wallin, & Shauffer, 2012). The paper purports to be a "review of literature," but it is a highly selective review. It draws policy implications that are draconian. Dozier et al. (2012) call for the abolition of all forms of residential care, a position consistent with that of Casey and the Lancet group. While scholars have a right to their ideological position, the broader view of the literature provided in this book shows that their position is not based on solid research evidence. What are the consequences?

First, the abolition of residential care would leave a significant group of children without a potentially life-changing option. They will be condemned to a life of unceasing instability as they move from one failing family situation to another, one foster family to another, perhaps with a short-term stay in a group home or two sprinkled in. Sibling groups that could be kept together in residential care will be separated. This is not speculation. Unstable foster care placements are common (e.g., Connell et al., 2006; Newton, Litrownik, & Landsverk, 2000). Breakdowns are processes, not isolated incidents (Bombach, Gabriel, & Stohler, 2018). When they occur, children and youth lose friends, school connections, and a sense of control over their own destiny (Unrau, Seita, & Putney, 2008). Moreover, in Britain, Clough (2005) found that among children and youth over five years of age in care, only 10% wanted to be adopted. Most wanted some contact with their families, often a grandparent, but did not want to live with their biological families (also see Attar-Schwartz & Huri, 2019). An unfortunate hierarchy of care, with residential care the last resort, has been created (Stuck, Small, & Ainsworth, 2000). It is not based on research evidence (McSherry, Fargas Malet, & Weatherall, 2016). From her work with former residents of the extremely deprived Romanian "orphanages," Neagu (2021) argues that while

> ...deinstitutionalisation is a global priority pushed by Western NGOs and international organisations...One key finding of the current study is that all types of placements have their challenges and they do not

> necessarily support a hierarchy of types of placement. The quality of care seemed to depend on the relationship children had with their carers regardless of the type of placement they were in.
>
> (p. 6)

Second, the calls for the abolition of residential care stigmatizes those who are in care. As Beker (2001) says, "…residential programs start out on the defensive, and to advocate for them is to make oneself vulnerable to the charge that his or her values are somehow outdated and/or otherwise flawed" (p. 444). Those who are currently in care are told that they are getting second-rate care. Those who are experiencing high-quality care generally know better, but there is no reason to lead them to believe that they are being harmed when they know they are not.

Third, perhaps the cruelest consequence of the blanket condemnation of residential care is that those who work with children and youth, often at great sacrifice, are stigmatized. They are sometimes unfairly accused of resisting the abolition of residential care because of "…a financial interest in the institution…" (Dozier et al., 2012, p. 16). I suspect that few people who are involved in providing the kind of high-quality care outlined in Chapter 6 are in it for the money. The work is physically and emotionally too demanding. This particular category of consequence has a strong odor of armchair analysis rather than a first-hand experience with actual caregivers.

Fourth, when the policy is to eliminate all residential care, there is little motivation to improve the existing care. This state of affairs is apparent in the subtitle of R. McCall's (2013) paper: *Can institutions be improved?: Should they*? If all residential care is inherently harmful, any attempts to improve it are misguided. If the evidence supported that inherent harmfulness, there would be no question about improving residential care. But, as we have seen, it does not. McCall was the leader of The St. Petersburg-USA Orphanage Research Team that found that improved care for infants and young children, including training caregivers to be more responsive and decreasing caregiver-child ratios, was related to developmental gains for children (The St. Petersburg-USA Orphanage Research Team, 2008). Yet, what by now is a long-held policy, one further exacerbated by the provisions of the Family First Prevention Services Act in the United States, is to make stays in residential care as short as possible. Social workers are pressured to remove the child or youth from residential care to other forms of care even when the residential care is demonstrably better for a particular child or youth and even preferred by the child or youth. Often what the child needs is a stable environment that allows them to build relationships with adults, peers, their schools, and their communities. Artificial time limits on residential care are often not in the best interests of the child. In countries where residential care is more highly esteemed, active improvements are being made (James et al., 2022). Where residential care is not respected, it is unlikely to receive the attention and resources its residents deserve (Anglin, Saint-Girons, & Trocmé,

2023). In countries where deinstitutionalization is ongoing, it is important that the best interests of children and youth are not eclipsed by simplistic dichotomies (e.g., Ramaswamy & Seshadri, 2020).

Fifth, blanket condemnation calls for the changing of the beliefs of individuals and organizations who have been "misled" into supporting residential care. Communities, families, and, especially donors, need to be "convinced" that they are aiding and abetting bad practice. Donors have been lured into supporting residential care "unaware of the harm that institutions cause" (Dozier et al., 2012, p. 16). "Gullible" donors have been led to believe they are helping children without parents and when visiting institutions, have been duped by the indiscriminate sociability of toddlers with poor attachments into thinking the children are being helped (the reference to indiscriminate sociability in the Dozier et al. paper betrays the overgeneralization from the infant research). There is no evidentiary basis for suggesting that supporters of high-quality residential care have been duped.

Finally, in the United States, the United Kingdom, and elsewhere, the condemnation of residential care has led to an absence of research support for studying residential care (Boel-Studt & Tobia, 2016; Whittaker, 2017; Whittaker et al., 2016). It is likely that there has been no federally funded research on residential care in the United States since the early years of research on the Teaching Family model over 50 years ago. Dozier et al. (2012) conclude that "All too frequently in the area of child welfare, programs are implemented that do not have an evidence base" (p. 18). Yet, it is the attitude toward residential care found in Dozier et al. itself that has made the kind of research Dozier and her colleagues call for un-fundable.

Proposition 4. There Is Ample Research That Supports the Use of Residential Care in the Array of Services for Children and Youth Who Need a Home

The research summarized in Chapter 4 shows that a blanket condemnation of residential care as ineffective and unalloyed support for foster care as an alternative is overly simplistic and unwarranted. Richard McKenzie, a highly respected economist, has provided unique data sets tapping into the lived experience of many former residents of children's homes. His work is rarely cited in the child welfare literature. We should not ignore it. Many adults who as children faced dire circumstances in mid-20th century America give much credit to those who took care of them at children's homes, the kinds of homes that today are considered last resorts. With McKenzie, we should ask: "Doesn't anyone (other than orphanage alumni) understand the value of permanence and stability to children?" (McKenzie, 1999, p. 18). The Duke Positive Outcomes for Orphans and OSCAR studies similarly support the contention that well designed and run residential care can have positive influences, even absent the rich resources of many children's homes in wealthier countries. Overall, when asked, those who have experienced good residential care frequently praise it (e.g., Kendrick, 2013; Neagu, 2021) and see foster care as a poor alternative.

Lee, Bright, Svoboda, Fakunmoju, and Barth's (2011) review of direct comparisons of residential care with alternatives gives weaker support for residential care but also does not show that it is somehow "inherently harmful." The pre-post only studies further question inherently negative effects even when dealing with juvenile offenders. Portwood, Boyd, and Murdock's (2016) study and Nixon and Henderson's (2022) study provide strong evidence of positive, not negative, change during residential care. Where residential care has become the option of "last resort," it often has become so because of a self-fulfilling prophecy in which a lack of attention to the quality of the care or the assignment of only the most troubled youth to care has led to poor outcomes (McNamara, 2023). Those in Stockholm who declared that the evidence of negative influences of residential care was indisputable should be disputed.

The literature on the effectiveness of foster care indicates that the simple set of equations residential care = bad, foster care/family = good, is simplistic indeed. As James and Roby (2019), commenting on the international scene (Ghana in particular) pose, the answer to "Does the reunification with family or other caregivers in the community (rather than remaining in the institution) actually serve the children's best interests? The answer it turns out, is perhaps more complex than previously conceptualized" (p. 316). Foster care is good when it is good. But often it is not good. Even adoption is far from perfect (Brodzinsky & Smith, 2019). An articulate young adult leaving care in the United Kingdom said:

> Many believe a family environment is a more suitable placement for a young person to grow up in. That may be the case for lots of young people and children in care, but not for all. Unfortunately, there seems to be a big push for foster care as residential care isn't viewed as an ideal option, more of a last resort if they can't find another suitable placement. That attitude needs to change, residential care homes work for a number of young people for reasons that are probably far too complicated than I can ever fully explain. But I do know that for me and a number of other young people, care homes were the BEST option, not the last resort option and they did some amazing work with us during our time there.
>
> (Narey, 2016, p. 5)

Thoburn (2016) states it succinctly:

> Although they will remain a minority, there are children and young people whose needs for a sense of permanence, and their wishes, can best be met by a longer stay placement in a children's home in which they can put down roots and which will provide continuity of relationships and a sense of community as they move into adult life.
>
> (p. 27)

Sometimes those who see the biological family as the *only* environment in which children can thrive have not been open to either the experience of children or the available research. Child-centered and family-centered are not always the same thing. Unqualified support for biological families can conflict with the best interests of the child. Similarly, belief in the importance of the least restrictive environment can be inconsistent with the best interests of the child when something else is what is needed. "Family-centered" and "least restrictive environments" are goods, but they are not unqualified goods. "It [residential care] can be the optimal placement for some young people whose experience of family and family-like placements has been associated with abuse, neglect, and placement breakdowns" (McNamara & Wall, 2023, p. 344).

Proposition 5. What Matters Most Is Not the Site at Which Care Occurs But the Quality of the Care a Child Receives

Perhaps what has struck me most in my review of this literature is that what matters is the quality of care a child or youth receives, not the setting in which it occurs (Boel-Studt & Tobia, 2016; Folman, 2009; Huynh et al., 2019; Knorth, Harder, Zandberg, & Kendrick, 2008; Neagu, 2021). As Folman (2009, p. 156) concludes: "It is *how* children live that matters, not *where* children live." Yet that simple fact seems to have been ignored in much of the child welfare literature.

Children need stability/continuity and resources. Yet, western child welfare systems seem constructed in a way to ensure disruption and change. The focus has been on "least restrictive environment" and "permanency" (in a family). The concept of least restrictive environment has been interpreted in terms of physical spaces and rules instead of psychological restraints. For children who have had consistently negative experiences in their families of origin and/or foster families, the freedom offered by a residential setting can provide the least restriction to being themselves that they have ever experienced. The legalistic use of least restrictive environment has a paradoxical outcome. The purported "permanency" provided by the system often is anything but permanent. Repeated placements, even ones with kind families doing their best to foster, mean no psychological permanence of place, peers, school, or relationships with adults.

The result is that children and youth who would benefit from a long-term placement in a children's home with a stable, caring staff, cannot have one. The strongly negative effects of moving from foster care home to foster care home is captured in the title of a study by Chambers et al. (2018): "It's just not right to move a kid that many times." Their respondents (adults who had been in the foster care system) echoed those of Unrau et al. (2008), who reported loss in multiple ways (also see Hyde & Kammerer, 2009). Good residential care is a better intervention than moving children and youth over and over. Thanks to the Family First Prevention Services Act, for a significant group of children and youth in the United States, stability and continuity may be less likely than it once was. Holmes et al. (2018) say it clearly:

> Studies within the field of child welfare show that it is not the individual versus group nature of the care environment but rather it is the quality of the care provided that affects outcomes. The nature of the engagement with the young people and the social interaction and activities in a placement make the difference.
>
> (Holmes et al., 2018, p. 215)

The quality of care has proven repeatedly to be more important than the type of care (Hermenau, Goessmann, Rygaard, Lindolt, & Hecker, 2017). The Danes have it right: "Children First" (Lausten, 2023).

Some scholars suggest that we do not know what constitutes quality in residential care. They say "nothing works" (e.g., Souverein, Van der Helm, & Stams, 2013). I believe from my review of the literature for Chapter 6 and what I know about research in child development that we *do* know what makes for quality care (also see Boel-Studt, Huefner, & Huang, 2019). First, Li and Julian (2012) have it right. What clearly matters to the success of any care are strong relationships (what they called the "secret ingredient" in successful interventions of all kinds) and long-term stability. In other words, children and youth need stable attachments, not multiple placements. They need positive relationships with trustworthy adults but also with supportive peers. Perhaps because of the infant/young child bias in the literature, those who believe children and youth can only thrive in families tend to forget that for the survival of the species, relationships with peers are eventually more important than relationships with family. Without them, the species would not survive. They need frequent opportunities to develop and exercise competencies and self-regulation and impulse controls (Cameron-Mathiassen, Leiper, Simpson, & McDermott, 2022). To do so, they need opportunities to be challenged in their educational, vocational, and recreational activities. They need to learn self-help and independent living skills. Compared to what happens even in the best of families, that all must be done more intentionally. Not surprising, these are just what is offered in the CARE and Teaching Family models.

On quality from an international perspective, Huynh et al. (2019, p. 8) say:

> Findings from this study underscore the role of key components of quality care on child psychosocial well-being. Importantly, child psychosocial well-being did not vary by residential vs. family-based care within levels of high- and low-quality care.

Also from an international perspective, Braitstein (2015) editorializes: "The evidence is mounting that at least in some places, institutional environments actually create family-like environments...there is nothing *necessary* about living in an institution that seems to be inherently bad for a child" (p. 331). Many promising programs are described in the recent *Revitalizing residential care for children and youth* volume (Whittaker, Holmes, del Valle, & James, 2023b). Examples include "No Wrong Door," a comprehensive approach to placement and treatment in England, "On the Way Home," a transition and aftercare program in the United States, "The Why Not? Trust" after care relationship program in Scotland, the "PLANEA" online training program for direct care workers in Spain, and the "KINGS" program for treating child and family trauma in the Netherlands. Residential care *should* be revitalized, not abandoned.

When the progressives called for foster care rather than orphanages at the White House Conference of 1909, surely, they did not imagine a foster care system where children would move constantly from one family to another. Nor could they have imagined that there would be foster families that grew to a size that approached the size of children's home cottages, but without the extra resources. They could not have imagined a system overwhelmed with family-less children and youth who spend many nights in the offices of social service workers or in motels, waiting for a placement, any placement, in a family. And, if they were truly progressive, they could not have imagined a system that pushed family reunification to the point that families were permanently broken up because parents could not get everything together fast enough to retain their parental rights.

Proposition 6. Residential Care Is Expensive. It Should Be

A surprising (to me) characteristic of the child welfare literature is the focus on cost as a disqualifier of residential care. In their letter to President Theodore Roosevelt, the conferees at the 1909 White House Conference on Dependent Children wrote: "Cheap care of children is ultimately enormously expensive…" (Hart, Butler, Mack, Folks, & West, 1909, p. 194). That has not changed. Certainly, an organization must be cognizant of cost effectiveness. Too often, however, the priority of expense seems to outweigh the best interests of the child. There is little doubt that residential care is more expensive than care in families in the short run (McCrae, Lee, Barth, & Rauktis, 2010). However, a long-term cost/benefit analysis can paint a different picture (Beker, 2001). The psychological costs of multiple foster placements or separation from siblings are a high price to pay (Cross, Koh, Rolock, & Eblen-Manning, 2013). If a child or youth can experience fewer damaging placements (Palmer, Ahn, Traube, Prindle, & Putnam-Hornstein, 2020), the costs of stabilizing them can be reduced substantially (Ringle Ingram & Thompson, 2010). Basing decisions about children and youth largely on economic terms is a violation of the principle of doing what is in the best interest of the child (Huefner, Ringle, Thompson, & Wilson, 2018) and the best interests of the communities they do and will live in. When residential care is part of an array of services in which organizations have multiple options, including various forms of foster care, adoption services, and independent living programs, decisions can be made about what is in the best interest of the child with cost as a secondary consideration.

In the United States, federal policy is that children should not face more than two placements before finding a permanent home. In California not that long ago, a majority (71%) faced more than that and a significant minority had a history of six to 20 placements (Malia, Quigley, Dowty, & Danjczek, 2008). A truism is that the most cost-effective placement is the one that is most effective—what is best for the child. Malia et al. (2008) used an apt medical analogy. Two aspirin and a morning call is the cheapest, least restrictive treatment for an appendicitis, but not in the best interest of the patient. Sometimes high-quality residential care provides the stability that in the long run is cheapest in fiscal and psychological costs (Boel-Studt & Tobia, 2016; Sunseri, 2005).

Proposition 7. The Conventional Wisdom Is Wrong, But What Do We Do before the Ideal Research Gets Here?

It is de rigueur to conclude we need more and better research. Of course, we could use the perfect randomized clinical trial of different forms of care, with large, representative groups, precise and meaningful measures of a broad range of psychological and neurological characteristics, a 20-year longitudinal design. That's all. In a research area plagued by methodological problems, that is what we need. It isn't going to happen. Too expensive. Too impractical. Takes too long. We live in an anti-residential care environment, without regard to evidence. Little knowledge is available on residential care in the United States in part because there has been a lack of interest on the part of policy makers and scholars for over 40 years and the private agencies who care about it only care to get rid of it (Courtney & Hughes-Iwaniec, 2009). Though not impossible (Boyd, Einbinder, Rauktis, & Portwood, 2007), it is difficult for small-scale agencies to do research.

We cannot wait for the perfect answer. So, what kind of research should be done? Perhaps more important than anything else, this research area cries out for an opening of the independent variable black box (Farmer, Wagner, Burns, & Murray, 2016; James, 2023; Knorth et al., 2008; Lee & Barth, 2011; Palareti & Berti, 2009). We need rich (and, in qualitative research jargon, "thick") descriptions of the interventions, whether they be different types of foster care or residential care (one good example can be found in Curtis, Alexander, and Lunghofer, 2001; and The St. Petersburg-USA Orphanage Research Team, 2005, provides another good model in their descriptions of Russian Baby Homes). We do not lack quantities of research. The mainstream child welfare journals are swollen to the point of distension. Yet, in the hundreds of articles I have read over the past few years, I can count on a hand or two the number that provide an adequate description of the program being examined (among the exceptions are those interventions like CARE and Teaching Family Model that have manualized training). Until we know better what the intervention is, discussions of outcomes and their causes are moot. Only then will we identify models of proven effectiveness that are replicable (Whittaker et al., 2016).

Along with Palareti and Berti (2009) and Little, Kohm, and Thompson (2005), also high on my list would be research about "fit." Who responds to what kind of intervention (Libby, Coen, Price, Silverman, & Orton, 2005)? For example, who is a candidate for foster care versus residential care? I have known too many youth in residential care who, when faced with yet another foster care placement ordered by a judge, will either undermine the new placement or simply run away. What developmental histories make adjustments, resiliency, or failure, more likely? And, not just what works, but why it does or does not work. I am not at all convinced that "family" is the answer to all the questions. Perhaps "family" as a set of biologically-related individuals should be replaced, as some sociologists have argued, with "home," a group of individuals with real psychological attachments (Kendrick, 2013; Mallett, 2004). "Who is my family?" is a question about relationships, not DNA. Mason and Tipper (2008) argue that family is a set of practices, not a biological entity or a social institution. We need ecologically complex research (Palareti & Berti, 2009).

I worry that there are real children and youth with real needs out there who are being shunted from placement to placement (including stops, often multiple stops, in their families of origin) while we wait for ideal research. The system envisioned by the Family First Prevention Services Act has not been working. I see no reason that it suddenly will begin to work because it has been legislated. The anti-residential care movement has momentum. Children, and especially youth, will be in families they know are not their family and whom they know they do not want to spend any length of time in. Before all the research can be done, I believe we need a very different line of investigation. We need a set of well-researched models that are replicable. Experts will need to take a very close look at these models and make judgments about their quality, effectiveness, and replicability. Folman (2009) asks:

> Isn't it time to recalculate what truly is "in the best interests of the child" and develop model programs, policies and procedures that enhance the placement experiences and adult outcomes of young people who grow up in the care of strangers?
>
> (p. 167)

Having a set of internationally recognized models could go a long way toward filling the gaps until the research is in.

Proposition 8. Everything Is More Complicated Than You'd Like to Think

Under the best possible circumstances, dealing with children and youth is complex. Trite, but true. Decisions about family dysfunction, child removal, entrance into care, and family reunification are embedded in broader issues of poverty, housing, joblessness and job training, divorce laws, child welfare laws, crime, health and addiction, racism, politics, and culture. As a further complication, the definitions and implications of all these issues change over time. Let me tell you about just one example I encountered while researching this book (much of this history is available in Jones, 1993; and Stuck et al., 2000). There is a long history in the United States of children being removed from their families because their single parent (typically a mother) is unable to provide for her children's basic needs. Before the Aid to Families with Dependent Children Act in the social legislation of the 1930s, poverty was the most likely reason why children ended up in institutions. Although the 1935 Social Security legislation led to significant declines in the "orphanage" census, poverty did not go away. Moreover, in the 1960s and 1970s a renewed concern with child neglect and abuse led to a new wave of child removals. Foster care of various sorts was needed. However, it was soon discovered that children were being "lost in the system." They tended to drift from foster family to foster family. New concerns for the health and safety of the child and what was called "permanency" came to the fore. The Adoption Assistance and Child Welfare Act of 1980 was designed to keep children from entering the foster care system and to make it easier, when that was impossible, to move toward the ending of parent rights and having the child adopted, thus attaining permanency for the child. The 1980 Act required that "reasonable efforts" be made at family reunification prior to ending parental rights and proceeding with adoption. Congress found that the move toward permanency was hampered by those "reasonable efforts." The Adoption and Safe Families Act of 1997 put more emphasis on the health and safety of the child, attenuated the "reasonable efforts," and sped up the moves toward permanency.

Wilhelm (2002) and Font, Sattler, and Gershoff (2018) argue that the elimination of the reasonable effort provision has led to premature termination of parental rights disproportionately among African American families. The terms used in the 1980 and 1997 laws, "reasonable efforts," "permanency," "abuse and neglect," and "reunification," all are ambiguous and therefore open to broad, subjective interpretation and misguided decision making. The rush to reunification may not provide enough time for families to be ready (Font et al., 2018), especially families whose children have experienced numerous placements (Carnochan, Lee, & Austin, 2013).

What does this have to do with residential care? If reunification of a family is to work, it takes time. Not two weeks or not even 18 months in many cases. For example, mothers with substance abuse issues often want to keep their children but struggle with their own problems, due to long histories of complex and difficult lives. In the absence of, and sometimes in the presence of, significant intervention and rehabilitation support, reunification can be difficult (Dare, Wilkinson, Karthigesu, Coall, & Marquis, 2023). Many high-quality residential care homes provide both respite from a dysfunctional family for the child and support services for the family. Residential care can (and currently often does) provide families with opportunities to heal. If the family is not salvageable, an extended period in residential care can provide the child with skills that make successful fostering or adoption more likely. All successful child-adult relationships depend on a proper fit in which the child sends off clear signals and the adult reads and responds in appropriate ways (Li and Julian's "active ingredient"). Neither the elimination of residential care nor the acceleration of parental rights terminations is going to help find that fit. Development is change in complexity. Simple equations like family is good, residential care is bad are too simple.

The shortcomings of the world's systems for dealing with children in need are many. Any form of childcare can be corrupted. Extreme environmental deprivation, child neglect and abuse, criminal trafficking, transactional foster care, confusion between poverty and neglect, premature termination of parental rights, practice without discernment, and many, many other problems need to be addressed. But Whittaker, Holmes, del Valle, and James (2023a, p. 4) are correct in their optimism: "...high-quality residential care, rigorously evaluated and connected to families and communities has a vital role to play in the future of child welfare systems." We need to see *all* children as gifts to be treasured, wherever they live. We need to act on their behalf with guarded regard for theory, ideology, or technique to make their lives better. We need to give them hope. Eliminating good residential care as an option for children and youth who need a safe, stable home solves no problem, meets no need, and does not serve the best interests of our children.

References

Ainsworth, F., & Hansen, P. (2005). A dream come true – No more residential care. A corrective note. *International Journal of Social Welfare*, *14*, 195–199. doi: 10.1111/j.1468-2397.2005.00359.x.

Alpert, L. T., & Meezan, W. (2012). Moving away from congregate care: One state's path to reform and lessons for the field. *Children and Youth Services Review*, *34*, 1519–1532. doi: 10.1016/j.childyouth.2012.04.003.

Anglin, J. P., Saint-Girons, M., & Trocmé, N. (2023). Residential care for children and youth in Canada. In J. K. Whittaker, L. Holmes, J. F. del Valle, & S. James (Eds.), *Revitalizing residential care for children and youth: Cross-national trends and challenges* (pp. 75–90). New York: Oxford University Press. doi: 10.1093/oso/9780197644300.003.0006.

Attar-Schwartz, S., & Huri, Y. (2019). Grandparental support and life satisfaction among adolescents in residential care. *Children and Youth Services Review*, *96*, 70–78. doi: 10.1016/j.childyouth.2018.11.033.

Beker, J. (2001). Back to the future: Effective residential group care and treatment for children and youth and the Fritz Redl Legacy. *Child & Youth Care Forum*, *30*, 443–455. doi: 10.1023/A:1015329501206.

Boel-Studt, S., Huefner, J. C., & Huang, H. (2019). The group care quality standards assessment: A framework for assessment, quality improvement, and effectiveness. *Children and Youth Services Review*, *105*, 104425. doi: 10.1016/j.childyouth.2019.104425.

Boel-Studt, S. M., & Tobia, L. (2016). A review of trends, research, and recommendations for strengthening the evidence-base and quality of residential group care. *Residential Treatment for Children & Youth*, *33*, 13–35. doi: 10.1080/0886571X.2016.1175995.

Bombach, C., Gabriel, T., & Stohler, R. (2018). Acknowledging the complexity of processes leading to foster care breakdown. *International Journal of Child, Youth and Family Studies*, *9*, 38–60. doi: 10.18357/ijcyfs92201818212.

Boyd, A. S., Einbinder, S. D., Rauktis, M. E., & Portwood, S. G. (2007). Building research capacity in residential treatment centers: An approach for empirical studies. *Child & Youth Care Forum*, *36*, 43–58. doi: 10.1007/s10566-006-9030-y.

Braitstein, P. (2015). Institutional care of children in low- and middle-income settings: Challenging the conventional wisdom of Oliver Twist. [Editorial]. *Global Health: Science and Practice*, *3*, 330–332. doi: 10.9745/GHSP-D-15-00228.

Brodzinsky, D., & Smith, S. L. (2019). Commentary: Understanding research, policy, and practice issues in adoption instability. *Research on Social Work Practice*, *29*, 185–194. doi: 10.1177/1049731518782647.

Cameron-Mathiassen, J., Leiper, J., Simpson, J., & McDermott, E. (2022). What was care like for me? A systematic review of the experiences of young people living in residential care. *Children and Youth Services Review*, *138*, 106524. doi: 10.1016/j.childyouth.2022.106524.

Carnochan, S., Lee, C., & Austin, M. J. (2013). Achieving timely reunification. *Journal of Evidence-Based Social Work*, *10*, 179–195. doi: 10.1080/15433714.2013.788948.

Chambers, R. M., Crutchfield, R. M., Willis, T. Y., Cuza, H. A., Otero, A., Goddu Harper, S. G., & Carmichael, H. (2018). "It's just not right to move a kid that many times": A qualitative study of how foster care alumni perceive placement moves. *Children and Youth Services Review*, *86*, 76–83. doi: 10.1016/j.childyouth.2018.01.028.

Child Welfare League of America (2005a). Position statement on residential services. Washington, DC: Author. Retrieved October 6, 2010, from http://www.cwla.org/programs/groupcare/rgcpositionstatement.pdf

Clough, R. (2005). Children in residence. In N. Axford, V. Berry, M. Little, & L. Morpeth (Eds.), *Forty years of research, policy and practice in children's services: A festschrift for Roger Bullock* (pp. 43–55). Oxford: Wiley-Blackwell.

Connell, C. M., Vanderploeg, J. J., Flaspohler, P., Katz, K. H., Saunders, L., & Tebes, J. K. (2006). Changes in placement among children in foster care: A longitudinal study of child and case influences. *Social Services Review*, *80*, 398–418. doi: 10.1086/505554.

Courtney, M. E., & Hughes-Heuring, D. (2009). Residential care in the United States of America: Past, present, and future. In M. E. Courtney & D. Iwaniec (Eds.), *Residential care of children: Comparative perspectives* (pp. 173–190). New York: Oxford Scholarship Online.

Cross, T. P., Koh, E., Rolock, N., & Eblen-Manning, J. (2013). Why do children experience multiple placement changes in foster care?: Content analysis on reasons for instability. *Journal of Public Child Welfare*, *7*, 39–58. doi: 10.1080/15548732.2013.751300.

Curtis, P. A., Alexander, G., & Lunghofer, L. A. (2001). A literature review comparing the outcomes of residential group care and therapeutic foster care. *Child and Adolescent Social Work Journal*, *18*, 377–392. doi: 10.1023/A:1012507407702.

Dare, J., Wilkinson, C., Karthigesu, S. P., Coall, D. A., & Marquis, R. (2023). Keeping the family: A socio-ecological perspective on the challenges of child removal and reunification for mothers who have experienced substance-related harms. *Children and Youth Services Review*, *145*, 106772. doi: 10.1016/j.childyouth.2022.106772.

Dozier, M., Kaufman, J., Kobak, R., O'Connor, T. G., Sagi-Schwartz A., Scott, S, … Zeanah, C. H. (2014). Consensus statement on group care for children and adolescents: A statement of Policy of the American Orthopsychiatric Association. *American Journal of Orthopsychiatry*, *84*, 219–225. doi: 10.1037/ort0000005.

Dozier, M., Zeanah, C. H., Wallin, A. R., & Shauffer, C. (2012). Institutional care for young children: Review of literature and policy implications. *Social Issues and Policy Review*, *6*, 1–25. doi: 10.1111/j.1751-2409.2011.01033.x.

Farmer, E. M. Z., Wagner, H. R., Burns, B. J., & Murray, M. (2016). Who goes where?: Exploring factors related to placement among group homes. *Journal of Emotional and Behavioral Disorders*, *24*, 54–63. doi: 10.1177/1063426615585082.

Ferguson, H. (2007). Abuse and looked after children as 'moral dirt': Child abuse and institutional care in historical perspective, *Journal of Social Policy, 36*, 123–139. doi:10.1017/S0047279406000407

Findley, M. G., Kikuta, K., & Denly, M. (2021). External validity. *Annual Review of Political Science*, *24*, 365–393. doi: 10.1146/annurev-polisci-041719-102556.

Folman, R. (2009). It is how children live that matters, not where children live. In W. K. Brown & J. R. Seita (Eds.), *Growing up in the care of strangers: The experiences, insights and recommendations of eleven former foster kids* (pp. 141–158). Tallahassee, FL: William Gladden Foundation Press.

Font, S. A., Sattler, K. M. P., & Gershoff, E. (2018). When home is still unsafe: From family reunification to foster care reentry. *Journal of Marriage and Family*, *80*, 1333–1343. doi: 10.1111/jomf.12499.

Goldman, P. S., Bakermans-Kranenburg, M. J., Bradford, B., Christopoulos, A., Ken, P. L. A., Cuthbert, C., … Sonuga-Barke, E. J. S. (2020). Institutionalisation and deinstitutionalisation of children 2: Policy and practice recommendations for global, national, and local actors. *Lancet Child and Adolescent Health*, *4*, 606–633. doi: 10.1016/S2352-4642(20)30060-2.

Gray, A. P., & Cote, W. (2019). Cultural connectedness protects mental health against the effect of historical trauma among Anishinabe young adults. *Public Health*, *176*, 77–81. doi: 10.1016/j.puhe.2018.12.003.

Hart, H. H., Butler, E. J., Mack, J. W., Folks, H., & West, J. E. (1909). Letter to the President of the United States embodying the conclusions of the Proceedings of the Conference on the Care of Dependent Children. In *Proceedings of the Conference on the Care of Dependent Children* (pp. 192–197). Washington, DC: Government Printing Office.

Hermenau, K., Goessmann, K., Rygaard, N. P., Landolt, M. A., & Hecker, T. (2017). Fostering child development by improving care quality: A systematic review of the effectiveness of structural interventions and caregiver trainings in institutional care. *Trauma, Violence, & Abuse*, *18*, 544–561. doi: 10.1177/1524838016641918.

Holmes, L., Connolly, C., Mortimer, E., & Hevesi, R. (2018). Residential group care as a last resort: Challenging the rhetoric. *Residential Treatment for Children & Youth*, *35*, 209–224. doi: 10.1080/0886571X.2018.1455562.

Huefner, J. C., Ringle, J. L., Thompson, R. W., & Wilson, F. A. (2018). Economic evaluation of residential length of stay and long-term outcomes. *Residential Treatment for Children and Youth*, *35*, 192–208. doi: 10.1080/0886571X.2018.1437375.

Huynh, H. V. (2019). Lessons learned from high-quality residential care centers around the world: A visual story. *International Journal on Child Maltreatment: Research, Policy and Practice*, 2, 99–116. doi: 10.1007/s42448-019-00018-5.

Huynh H. V., Limber, S. P., Gray, C. L., Thompson, M. P., Wasonga, A. I., Vann, V., ... Whetten, K. (2019). Factors affecting the psychosocial well-being of orphan and separated children in five low- and middle-income countries: Which is more important, quality of care or care setting? *PLoS ONE*, *14*(6): e0218100. doi: 10.1371/journal.pone.0218100.

Hyde, J., & Kammerer, N. (2009). Adolescents' perspectives on placement moves and congregate settings: Complex and cumulative instabilities in out-of-home care. *Children and Youth Services Review*, *31*, 265–273. doi: 10.1016/j.childyouth.2008.07.019.

James, S. (2011). What works in group care?—A structured review of treatment models for group homes and residential care. *Children and Youth Services Review*, *33*, 308–321. doi: 10.1016/j.childyouth.2010.09.014.

James, S. (2023). A cross-national comparison of residential care for children and youth: Conceptual and methodological foundations. In J. K. Whittaker, L. Holmes, J. F. del Valle, & S. James (Eds.), *Revitalizing residential care for children and youth: Cross-national trends and challenges* (pp. 25–40). New York: Oxford University Press. doi: 10.1093/oso/9780197644300.003.0003.

James, S. L., & Roby, J. L. (2019). Comparing reunified and residential care facility children's well being in Ghana: The role of hope. *Children and Youth Services Review*, *96*, 316–325. doi: 10.1016/j.childyouth.2018.12.001.

James, S., Wilczek, L., Kilian, J., Kallio, E. T., Bravo, A., del Valle, J. F., Formenti, L., Petrauskiene, A., Pivoriene, J., & Rigamonti, A. (2022). A comparative analysis of residential care: A five country multiple case design study. *Child & Youth Care Forum*, *51*, 1031–1062. doi: 10.1007/s10566-021-09666-6.

Jones, M. B. (1993). Decline of the American orphanage, 1941-1980. *Social Services Review*, *67*, 459–480. doi: 10.1086/603999.

Kendrick, A. (2013). Relations, relationships and relatedness: Residential child care and the family metaphor. *Child and Family Social Work*, *18*, 77–86. doi: 10.1111/cfs.12040.

Knorth, E. J., Harder, A. T., Zandberg, T., & Kendrick, A. J. (2008). Under one roof: A review and selective meta-analysis on the outcomes of residential child and youth care. *Children and Youth Services Review*, *30*, 123–140. doi: 10.1016/j.childyouth.2007.09.001.

Lausten, M. (2023). Residential care for children and youth in Denmark. In J. K. Whittaker, L. Holmes, J. F. del Valle, & S. James (Eds.), *Revitalizing residential care for children and youth: Cross-national trends and challenges* (pp. 225–238). New York: Oxford University Press. doi: 10.1093/oso/9780197644300.003.0016.

Lee, B. R., & Barth, R. P. (2011). Defining group care programs: An index of reporting standards. *Child & Youth Care Forum*, *40*, 253–266. doi: 10.1007/s10566-011-9143-9.

Lee, B. R., Bright, C. L., Svoboda, D. V., Fakunmoju, S., & Barth, R. P. (2011). Outcomes of group care for youth: A review of comparative studies. *Research on Social Work Practice*, *21*, 177–189. doi: 10.1177/1049731510386243.

Li, J., & Julian, M. M. (2012). Developmental relationships as the active ingredient: A unifying working hypothesis of '"what works"' across intervention settings. *American Journal of Orthopsychiatry*, *82*, 157–166. doi: 10.1111/j.1939-0025.2012.01151.x.

Libby, A. M., Coen, A. S., Price, D. A., Silverman, K., & Orton, H. D. (2005). Inside the black box: What constitutes a day in a residential treatment centre? *International Journal of Social Welfare*, *14*, 176–183. doi: 10.1111/j.1468-2397.2005.00357.x.

Little, M., Kohm, A., & Thompson, R. (2005). The impact of residential placement on child development: Research and policy implications. *International Journal of Social Welfare*, *14*, 200–209. doi: 10.1111/j.1468-2397.2005.00360.x.

Lucas, J. W. (2003). Theory-testing, generalization, and the problem of external validity. *Sociological Theory*, *21*, 236–253. doi: 10.1111/1467-9558.00187.

Macarov, D. (2008). Families versus institutions: A global view. *Social Development Issues*, *30*, 102–116. Retrieved from: https://web.p.ebscohost.com/ehost/pdfviewer/pdfviewer?vid=0&sid=2c02d5ad-b11e-4eb1-9c7b-cb8ed038b173%40redis.

Malia, M. G., Quigley, R., Dowty, G., & Daniczek, M. (2008). The historic role of residential group care. *Reclaiming Children and Youth*, *17*, 43–51. Retrieved from: https://www.proquest.com/docview/214193230?pq-origsite=summon.

Mallett, S. (2004). Understanding home: A critical review of the literature. *Sociological Review*, *52*, 62–89. doi: 10.1111/j.1467-954X.2004.00442.x.

Mason, J., & Tipper, B. (2008). Being related: How children define and create kinship. *Childhood*, *15*, 441–460. doi: 10.1177/09075682080972.

McCall, R. B. (2013). The consequences of early institutionalization: Can institutions be improved? Should they? *Child and Adolescent Mental Health*, *18*, 193–201. doi: 10.1111/camh.12025.

McCall, R. B., van IJzendoorn, M. H., Juffer, F., Groark, C. J., & Groza, V. K. (2011). Children without permanent parents: Research, practice, and policy. *Monographs of the Society for Research in Child Development*, *76*(4). doi: 10.1111/j.1540-5834.2011.00624.x.

McCrae, J. S., Lee, B. R., Barth, R. P., & Rauktis, M. E. (2010). Comparing three years of well-being outcomes for youth in group care and nonkinship foster care. *Child Welfare*, *89*, 229–249. PMID: 20857889.

McKenzie, R. B. (Ed.). (1999). *Rethinking orphanages for the 21st century*. Thousand Oaks, CA: Sage.

McNamara, P. (2023). The "New Era" in Victorian therapeutic residential care: A decade on. In J. K. Whittaker, L. Holmes, J. F. del Valle, & S. James (Eds.), *Revitalizing residential care for children and youth: Cross-national trends and challenges* (pp. 405–418). New York: Oxford University Press. doi: 10.1093/oso/9780197644300.003.0027.

McNamara, P., & Wall, S. (2023). Australian residential care: Creating opportunities for hope and healing. In J. K. Whittaker, L. Holmes, J. F. del Valle, & S. James (Eds.), *Revitalizing residential care for children and youth: Cross-national trends and challenges* (pp. 339–355). New York: Oxford University Press. doi: 10.1093/oso/9780197644300.003.0023.

McSherry, D., Fargas Malet, M., & Weatherall, K. (2016). Comparing long-term placements for young children in care: Does placement type really matter? *Children and Youth Services Review*, *69*, 56–66. doi: 10.1016/j.childyouth.2016.07.021.

Moriarty, F. M. (1999). The nation's child welfare problems as viewed from the bench. In R. B. McKenzie (Ed.), *Rethinking orphanages for the 21st century* (pp. 39–45). Thousand Oaks, CA: Sage.

Narey, M. (2016). *Residential care in England: Report of Sir Martin Narey's independent review of children's residential care*. London: Department for Education. Retrieved from: https://assets.publishing.service.gov.uk/government/uploads/

system/uploads/attachment_data/file/534560/Residential-Care-in-England-Sir-Martin-Narey-July-2016.pdf.

Neagu, M. (2021). *Voices from the silent cradles: Life histories of Romania's looked after children*. Bristol: Policy Press.

Newton, R. R., Litrownik, A. J., & Landsverk, J. A. (2000). Children and youth in foster care: Disentangling the relationship between problem behaviors and number of placements. *Child Abuse & Neglect*, *24*, 1363–1374. doi: 10.1016/S0145-2134(00)00189-7.

Nixon, C., & Henderson, G. (2022). How is the provision of residential care to children under the age of 12 associated with changes in children's behaviour and mental wellbeing? *Scottish Journal of Residential Child Care*, *21*(1). Retrieved from: https://strathprints.strath.ac.uk/84133/1/Nixon_Henderson_SJRCC_2022_How_is_the_provision_of_residential_care.pdf.

Palareti, L., & Berti, C. (2009). Different ecological perspectives for evaluating residential care outcomes: Which window for the black box? *Children and Youth Services Review*, *31*, 1080–1085. doi: 10.1016/j.childyouth.2009.07.011.

Palmer, L., Ahn, E., Traube, D., Prindle, J., & Putnam-Hornstein, E. (2020). Correlates of entry into congregate care among a cohort of California foster youth. *Children and Youth Services Review*, *110*, 104772. doi: 10.1016/j.childyouth.2020.104772.

Portwood, S. G., Boyd, A. S., & Murdock, T. B. (2016). Implementation of a program of outcomes research in residential care settings: Outcomes for children and youth. *Child & Youth Care Forum*, *45*, 393–407. doi: 10.1007/s10566-015-9337-7.

Ramaswamy, S., & Seshadri, S. (2020). The deinstitutionalisation debate in India: Throwing the baby out with the bathwater? *Scottish Journal of Residential Care*, *19*(2). Retrieved from: https://www.celcis.org/application/files/2816/2306/7079/2020_Vol_19_No_2_Ramaswamy_S_The_Deinstitutionalisation_Debate_in_India.pdf.

Ringle, J. L., Ingram, S. D., & Thompson, R. W. (2010). The association between length of stay in residential care and educational achievement: Results from 5- and 16-year follow-up studies. *Children and Youth Services Review*, *32*, 974–980. doi: 10.1016/j.childyouth.2010.03.022.

Rogoff, B., Dahl, A., & Callanan, M. (2018). The importance of understanding children's lived experience. *Developmental Review*, *50*, 5–15. doi: 10.1016/j.dr.2018.05.006.

Sherr, L., Roberts, K. J., & Gandhi, N. (2017). Child violence experiences in institutionalized/orphanage care. *Psychology, Health & Medicine*, 22, 31–57. doi: 10.1080/13548506.2016.1271951.

Smith, M. (2010). Victim narratives of historical abuse in residential child care do we really know what we think we know? *Qualitative Social Work*, 9, 303–320. doi: 10.1177/147332501036781.

Souverein, F. A., Van der Helm, G. H. P., & Stams, G. J. J. M. (2013). 'Nothing works' in secure residential youth care? *Children and Youth Services Review*, *35*, 1941–1945. doi: 10.1016/j.childyouth.2013.09.010.

Stuck, E. N., Small, R. W., & Ainsworth, F. (2000). Questioning the continuum of care: Toward a reconceptualization of child welfare services. *Residential Treatment for Children & Youth*, *17*, 79–92. doi: 10.1300/J007v17n03_12.

Sunseri, P. A. (2005). Children referred to residential care: Reducing multiple placements managing costs and improving treatment outcomes. *Residential Treatment for Children & Youth*, 22, 55–66. doi: 10.1300/J007v22n03_04.

The St. Petersburg-USA Orphanage Research Team. (2005). Characteristics of children, caregivers, and orphanages for young children in St. Petersburg, Russian Federation. *Journal of Applied Developmental Psychology*, *26*, 477–506. doi: 10.1016/j.appdev.2005.06.002.

The St. Petersburg-USA Orphanage Research Team. (2008). The effects of early social-emotional and relationship experience on the development of young orphanage children. *Monographs of the Society for Research in Child Development*, *73*(3). doi: 10.1002/9781444309683.

Thoburn, J. (2016). Residential care as a permanence option for young people needing longer-term care. *Children and Youth Services Review*, *69*, 19–28. doi: 10.1016/j.childyouth.2016.07.020.

Unrau, Y. A., Seita, J. R., & Putney, K. S. (2008). Former foster youth remember multiple placement moves: A journey of loss and hope. *Children and Youth Services Review*, *30*, 1256–1266. doi: 10.1016/j.childyouth.2008.03.010.

van IJzendoorn, M. H., Bakermans-Kranenburg, M., Duchinsky, R., Fox, N. A., Goldman, P. S., Gunnar, M. R., ... Sonuga-Barke, E. J. S. (2020). Institutionalisation and deinstitutionalisation of children 1: A systematic and integrative review of evidence regarding effects on development. *Lancet Psychiatry*, *4*, 1–18. doi: 10.1016/S2215-0366(19)30399-2.

van IJzendoorn, M. H., Palacios, J., Sonuga-Barke, E. J. S., Gunnar, M. R., Vorria, P., McCall, R. B., Le Mare, L., Bakermans-Kranenburg, M., Dobrova-Krol, N. A., & Juffer, F. (2011). Children in institutional care: Delayed development and resilience. In R. B. McCall, M. H. van IJzendoorn, F. Juffer, C. J. Groark, & Groza, V. K. (Eds.). Children without permanent parents: Research, practice, and policy. *Monographs of the Society for Research in Child Development*, *76*(4), 8–30. doi:10.1111/j.1540-5834.2011.00626.x

Whittaker, J. K. (2017). Pathways to evidence-based practice in therapeutic residential care: A commentary. *Journal of Emotional and Behavioral Disorders*, *25*, 57–61. doi: 10.1177/1063426616686345.

Whittaker, J. K., Holmes, L., del Valle, J. F., Ainsworth, F., Andreassen, T., Anglin, J., ... Zeira, A. (2016). Therapeutic residential care for children and youth: A consensus statement of the International Work Group on Therapeutic Care. *Residential Treatment for Children & Youth*, *33*, 89–106. doi: 10.1080/0886571X.2016.1215755.

Whittaker, J. K., Holmes, L., del Valle, J. F., & James, S. (2023a). Residential care for children and youth in a cross-national perspective. In J. K. Whittaker, L. Holmes, J. F. del Valle, & S. James (Eds.), *Revitalizing residential care for children and youth: Cross-national trends and challenges* (pp. 3–15). New York: Oxford University Press. doi: 10.1093/oso/9780197644300.003.0001.

Whittaker, J. K., Holmes, L., del Valle, J. F., & James, S. (Eds.). (2023b). *Revitalizing residential care for children and youth: Cross-national trends and challenges*. New York: Oxford University Press.

Wilhelm, P. A. (2002). Permanency at what cost?: Five years of imprudence under the Adoption and Safe Families Act of 1997. *Notre Dame Journal of Law, Ethics and Public Policy*, *16*(2), Article 15. Retrieved from: https://scholarship.law.nd.edu/ndjlepp/vol16/iss2/15.

Index

FSC
www.fsc.org
MIX
Papier | Fördert
gute Waldnutzung
FSC® C083411

Kolibri 360 GmbH
Ferdinand-Jühlke-Straße 7
99095 Erfurt, Deutschland
produktsicherheit@kolibri360.de